Paging Doctor A

Paging Doctor A

Continuing Stories from a Country Doctor

by

Jimmie Ashcraft, M.D.

First published by Dog Ear Publishing
4011 Vincennes Rd
Indianapolis, IN 46268
www.dogearpublishing.net

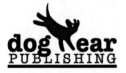

ISBN: 978-1-4575-4672-3

This book is printed on acid-free paper.

Printed in the United States of America

Original cover design by David Ashcraft

For
my children and grandchildren

"Promise me you'll always remember:
you're braver than you believe,
and stronger than you seem,
and smarter than you think."

Christopher Robin to Pooh

and always

Kay

Contents

A Tribute to Doctor A

Lyrics by Peggy Kopp, RN
Performed by the nursing staff from Sidney Health Center
at Dr. Ashcraft's retirement event 6/3/2001

Melody from *You've Got a Friend* by Carole King

When the day is long
And you need some good advice
And nothin' nothin' is going right
We dial the phone and call on you
And soon you will be here
To manage the crisis anytime day or night
We just call out your name...."Dr. Ashcraft to the delivery
room"
and we know wherever you are..."Dr. Ashcraft ER STAT"
You'll come runnin' to help us again and again
Winter, spring, summer or fall
All we have to do is call
And you'll be there
Doctor Ashcraft, jack of all trades
You treat all ailments and deliver babes
Asthmatics and heart attacks
Took out appendixes and fixed sore backs
Now retiring to a new phase
We hope you enjoy your lazy days
Good luck we say and now we're blue
Doctor Ashcraft we will miss you.

Melody from *The Candy Man*

Who can take a tractor
Use it for therapy
Drive it in the field to make hay or gardening
Dr. A can, Dr. A can

Who can take a basement
Turn it into a dream
With pain and a walking track
Success we've clearly seen
Dr. A can, Dr. A can

Building our community
Giving of your time
Dollars and cents

Building a track to run on
A fitness center
A baseball diamond
Giving of your love
Making it possible for young minds to learn
Giving a scholarship for children
Giving of yourself to us
We never will forget

Author's Preface

Over fifty years ago I was a young boy from a poor family with a burning desire of becoming a doctor someday so I could help people. All children have dreams about what they would like to be when they grow up, but few achieve them. I was one of the lucky ones. With the help of many and a lot of good luck I became a doctor and practiced medicine in rural Montana. Soon after I started my medical practice in Sidney, Montana, I told people that I was already an anachronism in my own time. I had the good fortune of being able to practice as a generalist family physician in an era of increasing specialization. This achievement was testimony to the excellence of my teachers, mentors, colleagues, training programs and my patients.

This retrospective offers more true stories about my life in medicine as a country doctor. I have done my best to portray the episodes as accurately as my memory and records would allow. Except for a select few, the names of individuals, my patients, their families, and my colleagues are changed to maintain confidentiality. Details that might identify certain people or places have been modified. The internet notations in the bibliography are accurate at the time of my research, but because the internet is ever changing, they may have changed since publication. Although others have reviewed my text and made suggestions, I am the final editor of the text and any errors are mine.

Acknowledgements

I never could have practiced medicine without magnificent teachers, mentors, and colleagues along the way. To them I owe my perpetual gratitude.

The hospital and nursing home personnel in Sidney, Montana, especially the nursing and laboratory staffs, taught me more than they will ever know about how to be a doc in a small town.

Without people willing to allow me the privilege of caring for them for over four decades there could be no books to tell their stories. I thank every one of them.

Mary and Richard Woods deserve a big thank-you. They took the time to read and reread the manuscript to help me simplify the language making the book more readable. I hope I succeeded in employing their concepts.

My children Jennifer, Becky, and David each played a significant role in making this fourth book possible.

Finally, my wife Kay read the text over and over again making important edits and suggestions. Her input and support, as always, was invaluable.

"It makes one's blood boil to think that there are sent out year-by-year scores of men called doctors, who have never attended a case of labor, and were utterly ignorant of the ordinary everyday diseases which they may be called upon to treat … is it to be wondered … that there is a widespread distrust in the public of a professional education, and that quacks, charlatans, and impostors possess the land?"

William Osler, "Licensed to Practice," May 11, 1889

Introduction

In 1904 a famous and legendary physician named Sir William Osler counseled doctors to *"Live a simple and temperate life, that you may give all your powers to your profession. Medicine is a jealous mistress; she will be satisfied with no less."* Unlike this famous advice, most physicians do not live a simple life. The demands by patients, hospitals, communities, political groups, and others for a doctor's time can be extraordinary. As a young boy Dr. Osler's mistress seduced me, and I have had a lifelong affair with her.

The book's title, *Paging Dr. A*, relates to the many ways I was summoned or contacted over the years. A phone ringing, or a pager beeping, or a nurse having a hunch about a patient, or a sheriff coming to my home in the middle of the night all requested my help. I learned that someone waving at me in a crowd, a pat on my back, or a note written on a scrap of paper could also be asking for my assistance with a medical problem or to give a presentation to educate others. With time and experience, I learned that a person's appearance and body language often communicated a better medical history than the spoken word.

This retrospective presents more true stories about my journey through fifty years of medicine. Some stories have extended notes inserted into the text to give the reader clarity about certain topics. Some stories contain "Food For Thought" topics. Like the stories in my other books, *Reflections of a Country Doctor*, *The Next Prescription*, and *Side Effects*, some are silly, some are sad, some will make you happy, and some might make you mad.

I hope you enjoy this portion of my life's journey in medicine.

A Bump in the Road

In 1968 I was a nineteen-year-old college student entering spring term and training for the upcoming outdoor track season. On Wednesday I had personal best times in my training sessions. Early Friday morning I was awakened by sweats, shaking chills, and excruciating pain in the groin area of both legs with severe lower back pain to the point I was unable to walk. After overcoming considerable reluctance from my mother, I was taken to the hospital emergency room where the doctor diagnosed strained leg muscles and sent me home with instructions to take a hot bath several times a day. The doctor failed to notice, and did not inform my mother, that I had a fever of 102°. My mother and I returned home and tried to follow the doctor's orders.

Early the next morning the pain worsened. Barely able to move my legs, I was having sweats and chills. Following the emergency room physician's instructions, my mother managed to get me into the bathtub for a warm bath, but the pain became so severe that I was unable to move. After I pleaded with my mother, she summoned an ambulance. The ambulance technicians had to lift me out of the bathtub because I could not move my legs.

By the time the ambulance got me to the hospital emergency room, I was delirious and apparently incoherent when Dr. George Brosius, an internal medicine specialist, came to evaluate me. My temperature had risen to 104°, and my blood pressure was dropping; I was going into shock caused by an infection. Within a short period of time X-rays were taken of my chest, pelvis, and back. A radiologic procedure called an intravenous pyelogram, or IVP, during which a contrast dye is injected into a vein before multiple x-rays are taken of the kidneys and the urinary system was performed. Multiple tests and samples were obtained from my blood, urine, nose, throat, and prostate to culture for bacteria. After all the tests were completed I was given multiple antibiotics until the doctors could figure out what was making me sick.

I was in and out of consciousness for the first day. The nurses administered large doses of a narcotic pain medicine and infused me with large volumes of intravenous fluids to maintain my blood pressure. On the morning of the third day I recall that Dr. Brcsius came in to talk with me since I hadn't been able to give him much of a history. After our conversation he told me he could find no good reason why I should become so full of infection. Earlier while I was in the emergency room, Dr. Brosius had requested consultation opinions from two of his partners, Dr. Sterling, an orthopedic surgeon, and Dr. Hagelman, a urologist. They too were puzzled by my illness.

That evening while making his rounds, Dr. Brosius informed me that the lab had discovered I was infected with a bad bacteria called Staphylococcus Aureus, and it was resistant to the usual penicillin antibiotics. Fortunately, a brand new antibiotic named Staphcillin[6] seemed to be working against the penicillin-resistant bacterium, and the doctor was going to start the medicine that evening. Unfortunately, the antibiotic had to be given into the muscle with an injection every four hours. The course of treatment would conclude after one hundred injections. I really didn't have much to say as he left the room. Throughout this ordeal I received potent pain medication and antibiotic injections every four hours.

Microbes such as the one that infected me are quite adept at change and within a few decades of excessive and often indiscriminate antibiotic use, a penicillin resistant germ, nicknamed MRSA (Methicillin-Resistant Staphylococcus Aureus), emerged and became prevalent in many hospitals.[7] By 2015, doctors could only wish that they had to deal with MRSA alone. As the good germs were eliminated by antibiotics over the decades, worse germs emerged that were resistant to just about everything in our pharmaceutical bag of microbe killers.

The next morning Dr. Hagelman came in early before surgery. He informed me that he was going to perform a rectal exam to massage my infected prostate gland. He said he had performed this procedure three times already when I was delirious and quipped that I probably didn't remember. I agreed that I did not remember the examination. Dr. Hagelman vigorously massaged my prostate with his index finger to remove as much pus and fluid as he could manually. He told me that my prostate was infected and that antibiotics did not kill germs very well in the prostate. He also told me that to cure an infected prostate it had to be drained and the only way to do that was with a vigorous massage. Dr. Hagelman asked the nurse if I had received my latest dose of pain medication because the procedure was going to be painful and he apologized in advance for the suffering he was going to inflict. Painful did not even come close to describing the discomfort. Not only did I have severe pain in the muscles of both legs but also I now had severe pain in the crotch.

Before leaving, Dr. Hagelman told me that the IVP x-rays of my kidneys revealed that everything was swollen, distorted, and stretched out from the infection. Reassuring me that they were now on top of my problem and knowing that it was going to take about three weeks to get the infection under control, the doctor urged me to be patient.

Soon after Dr. Hagelman left the room, Dr. Sterling came to visit. He told me it was nice to see me when I was coherent. As I was lying in the bed he gently touched the inner parts of my thighs to try to discern the location of most of my leg pain. Just a touch of his hand on the skin of my legs was more than I could tolerate. He found that because of the pain I could not bend my legs at the knees or the hips. When he tried to stand me up to walk, I collapsed because my legs would not support me. Dr. Sterling told me he wasn't really sure what was wrong with my muscles except that they appeared to be infected for reasons unknown to him. He assured me that Dr. Brosius had me on the right medicines and I would get better. He too asked me to be patient.

I really didn't know what I was going to do except be patient since I could barely roll over in bed. Going to the bathroom was almost impossible and embarrassing for a shy nineteen-year-old boy surrounded by female nurses.

Dr. Brosius faithfully made morning and evening visits even on weekends for about twenty days. Dr. Sterling came by about every other day to evaluate my progress in walking and to order physical therapy until the end of my hospital stay. Dr. Hagelman came by every morning at the same time, about fifteen minutes after I had received a pain medication shot in advance to minimize the pain that he was going to produce with his prostate massage. Dr. Hagelman would always apologize in advance and then proceed to massage my gland for seventeen consecutive mornings. Late in the evening on the 17th day Dr. Hagelman came into my room to tell me that my prostate fluid was now clear enough so that he didn't have to mash on my prostate anymore while I was in the hospital. I could have kissed him. I was beginning to think his index finger was a yard long.

My temperature normalized on about the twelfth day, and I was finally able to get up and walk to the bathroom without collapsing with the minimal assistance of two people.

On the eighteenth hospital day Dr. Brosius happily pronounced that I had received my one hundred injections of antibiotics. My repeat cultures were free of the germs, and I could be converted to oral antibiotics for another month of treatment. During the same time I had received an additional one hundred injections of pain medication. My butt was so sore that I had to sleep on my abdomen. I would come to know some of the hospital nurses by their first names because they took care of me most of the time. I learned which nurses gave reasonably painless injections, especially during the night shift, and when the student nurses were being trained to give injections.

In time, if antibiotics were to be given for the long-term or before surgeries, an intravenous route was used. Single doses of intra-muscular antibiotics would be reserved for special circumstances in an outpatient clinic. There were several good reasons for this change. First, if an allergic reaction to the medication occurred, there would not be a deposit of the medication in a muscle that could perpetuate the adverse reaction. Second, studies revealed that newer oral preparations of antibiotics were usually just as effective as injections. Finally, pills are easily dispensed by a pharmacy, are generally cheaper to administer, and don't hurt.

A generation later the narcotic pain medication given to me named Demerol was determined to have too many adverse reactions with other medications and was for the most part eliminated for general use. It was replaced with more potent narcotic pain medications with the names of morphine, hydromorphone, and oxycodone. Unfortunately, when some of these potent pain medications became available in tablet form, they caused an entirely new set of problems with drug addiction and illicit drug trafficking providing yet another example of the rule of unintended consequences.

Forty years later, having the same nurses care for a patient over multiple days would be unusual. Having a personal doctor care for his patient in the hospital would be a rare event at the onset of the twenty-first century with the introduction of the hospitalist, a physician specializing in hospital inpatient care.[8] Often the primary physician is no longer allowed in the hospital because it contends that hospitalist care is more efficient with better outcomes. I am not convinced. Medical care by its very nature is a personal, inefficient endeavor, and frankly, the hospitalist system is about as impersonal as it gets. It seems to me that the hospitalists are more concerned about data than about patients. As Sergeant Joe Friday from the television program *Dragnet* used to say, "Just the facts ma'am, just the facts." The bottom line for hospitals' use of hospitalists supposedly is better efficiency and higher quality patient care. Patients do stay in the hospital less time under a hospitalist's care. Unfortunately, the duties previously provided by hospital nurses are now performed by family members or in alternate care facilities. Supposedly, this equates financially to a better bottom line for the hospital. I am not sure about the higher quality care.

At the end of my twentieth hospital day I went home on crutches which I discarded a week or so later. For several years afterward I had frequent nightmares about my experience, especially about the pain and inability to walk. Three years later while I was in medical school I was finally able to run without pain in my legs. I still re-live this experience occasionally in my dreams half a century later.

At the same time of this hospital adventure I had a rash on my skin that had been present since I was thirteen years old and was thought to be no more than a mild irritation by the local dermatologist. Sometime later during my medical training I would learn that the rash was a rare form of skin cancer called mycosis fungoides (later to be renamed cutaneous T-cell lymphoma), which was usually found in old people, not teenagers.[9,10] Additionally I learned that the number one reason for people to die with this skin disease is a systemic bacterial infection caused by the same germ that infected me. The mystery for my severe infection was finally solved.

As I was writing this story almost forty-eight years later, I learned that Doctor George Brosius was still alive. I called him just after New Year's Day in 2016, asked if he remembered me at all, and arranged an appointment. At the meeting Dr. Brosius appeared much like I remembered him only older with stooped shoulders. He was now ninety-three years old and had practiced internal medicine in Billings, Montana, until he retired at age seventy-eight. Dr. Brosius admitted that he did not recall my case, but he did remember my name for some reason. After I gave him a few highlights of my clinical presentation at our first meeting in the hospital emergency room in the spring of 1968, Dr. Brosius recalled that I was a very sick lad indeed. After some thought he added that he and his partners were puzzled about my illness and not sure I would survive.

I gave Dr. Brosius my three books as a gift to remind him that his efforts helping a sick young college student decades before paid many dividends.

Emergency Department

Medical school started in the fall of 1970 at the University of Oregon Medical School in Portland, Oregon. My first few days were exhilarating; our new class of students would be doctors in four years. Within a short time, however, the initial exhilaration transformed into work, a lot of work. Lectures started at 8 a.m. every morning and concluded every afternoon about 5 p.m. Then another three to four hours of reading and studying continued after supper. On the weekends students tried to catch up on the studying they did not have time to complete during the week. After about a month or so of this regimen most of us settled into a rigorous eighty to one hundred hour workweek of studying anatomy, physiology, biochemistry, and other subjects. In the few remaining free hours during the week each student found ways to unwind. I wandered out into the patient care areas of the medical school complex to get energized. With just a few weeks of basic sciences study under my belt I decided to venture down to the hospital on a Friday night just to see what I could observe.

My first foray into clinical medicine was in Portland's Mult-nomah County Hospital emergency room. I introduced myself as a medical student to the clerk at the front desk and requested the opportunity to observe. The woman at the desk raised her arm with a pointed finger and told me to talk to the nurse a short distance away. I walked over to meet a short, stocky middle-aged woman in a white nursing uniform who was wearing a small white nursing cap. Printed on her name tag was Elizabeth Murphy, RN Supervisor. I introduced myself as a medical student who wanted to observe. Politely Mrs. Murphy introduced herself as the charge nurse for the evening, welcomed me to the emergency department, and asked me to stand near a certain wall until she could introduce me to the emergency room surgery resident on duty.

Within a short time I was directed to the physician's room where I met Doctor Wayne, the surgery intern on duty. My job was to follow him that first evening to see what I could pick up without getting in his way. Doctor Wayne's only request was that I stand aside during an acute emergency. He gave me instructions on which neutral corner of the emergency room to occupy saying, "You don't know anything, and your job is to observe."

I quickly noted that the person in command was not the doctor but the emergency room charge nurse, Mrs. Murphy. She controlled what patients were seen, when they were seen, and who saw them, a system called triage. She also determined where curious medical students like me could stand so they did not mess up the smooth operation of the emergency room.

The county hospital emergency department was a hospital's peacetime equivalent to the television program *M*A*S*H 4077* with the medical student like me being placed in the role of a doctor such as Hawkeye Pierce, MD, or Trapper John, MD. In reality, the inexperienced medical student is much more like Radar O'Reilly, the lowly clerk. He wears a white coat, but he doesn't have a clue about what's going on. Unfortunately, there is no director to yell, "Cut!" and cease the action at any point in time. I found the emergency room in the county hospital to be a continuously running 24-hour reality show where real people were the actors, some with serious problems who displayed genuine blood, guts, and gore.

I soon learned that a caregiver's survival in the emergency room required not questioning an exhausted, distraught mother who brought her sick child with a runny nose and sore throat to the emergency room at midnight. The woman's child had been sick for almost two weeks with the same symptoms, and she was tired of it.

I watched Mrs. Murphy attempt to triage patients by their complaints even when they were uncooperative. Drunks, drug addicts, and vagrants pose a most difficult challenge to the emergency worker when he or she tries to get a simple history and the patient has difficulty answering a few basic questions such as, "What is your name?" or "Where do you live?" However, a pleasant drunk singing the *Sound of Music* and claiming to be Marco Polo can be a pleasure to care for compared to the defiant abusive patient on drugs who refuses to give out any information about who she is, or why she's in the emergency room.

I was observing a disheveled man in filthy clothes with sores all over his face walk up to the admission desk. Before the clerk could get the man's name Mrs. Murphy called out and had an orderly take the man immediately to the delousing tank. She told the orderly to bag the man's clothes and throw them in the garbage. She then asked a nursing aide to find the man some clean clothes from the closet of clothing donated by the Salvation Army. Mrs. Murphy turned toward me and told me that the man was a drug addict, alcoholic, lived under a local bridge, and was a frequent flyer (visitor) to the emergency department. She told me that fleas and lice caused the sores on his face, and she wanted to kill the bugs before everyone in the emergency room got infected.

A favorite in the emergency room this night was the parent-child team where the child had a pain somewhere, and the parent was the real pain. The mom tells the doctor how sick her child is, and she knows that a bursting appendix is causing her child's lower abdominal pain. All the while, the child appears be perfectly content and certainly is able to give you a history about all the junk food that he had eaten several hours before, if the parent would allow the child to speak.

I soon appreciated Mrs. Murphy's admonition, "Expect the unexpected." No task, and I do mean no task, is too awesome or too ridiculous for the emergency room nurses or doctors to manage. Removing foreign objects from human bodies was all too common. Removing contact lenses and delousing hair, bodies, and clothing are nothing compared to the array of objects that are removed from the bodies of a variety of sexual adventurers on drugs. From retrieving light bulbs from the rectum to extracting hair curlers from the vagina, I soon learned to expect the unexpected.

Like many popular nightspots, the emergency department seemed to attract large weekend crowds, especially during the spring and summer months when would-be star athletes in their youth still sought the thrills of victory but more often experienced the agonies of their defeats. All too often the young doctor was treated to the repetitive play-by-play description of what happened to the star athlete and how things could have turned out differently only if....

Trying to decide who gets what place in the treatment queue is a daunting task for the charge nurse as well as an especially challenging duty for the young doctor to learn. The value of the experience of observing a skilled ER charge nurse triaging patients was priceless. Emergency department patients enjoy vying for position and are more than willing to tell you how they are sicker than the person in front of them. The more alcohol the patients have consumed always ups the ante on their personal triage scoreboards. One such patient started the bidding for position with, "The cuts all over my body are from a butcher knife!"

His best drinking buddy slurs back with, "Well, I was blasted by a shotgun at ten feet! Look at the holes in my belly."

A third fellow joins in with, "That's nothing! I just got blown up in a building downtown, and I almost died!" The real story was that they were all in a fight at a local pub, and the bouncer pummeled them severely.

From a far corner of the waiting room the mother with the child who still had a bellyache shouted out something like, "My child's appendix is going to rupture pretty soon, and you all are going to pay for it!"

Finally, there is the patient who ran into the emergency room and left his car running double-parked in a tow away zone. He sees a young medical student (me) in a short white coat believing that I am a person of responsibility. He confronts me, demands being seen right away because his car's in a tow away zone, and then sharply asks, "Do you know who I am?" The man has no idea that a short white coat in a medical school hospital just means medical student who knows nothing.

Before I could say a word, Mrs. Murphy, who was standing nearby and heard the conversation, interrupted with, "No, sir, I do not know who you are or who you think you are. I do know that you are still standing and talking, so please tell me your name so I can put you on the non-emergency waiting list. A doctor will see you when he can. By the way, you might want to park your car first because the tow truck is getting ready to haul it away — at your expense."

Doctor Wayne called out from across the emergency room and motioned for me to come to the trauma room. When I arrived at the assigned area, he informed me that multiple auto accidents had occurred on Interstate 80 east of Portland, ambulances were transporting perhaps fourteen patients to the Multnomah County emergency department, and they were to start arriving in a few minutes. Dr. Wayne pointed to my neutral corner in the trauma room where I could observe the action. I soon learned that at the county hospital emergency room any able-bodied person wearing a white coat was expected to be doing something useful.

In preparation for the arrival of multiple patients, the nursing personnel prepared multiple bottles of intravenous fluid solution and hung them all in a row so time would not be wasted. When the patients started to arrive the entire scene was controlled pandemonium with Mrs. Murphy orchestrating all the action. Despite the screaming and yelling of patients and the orderly commands from the charge nurse and Doctor Wayne, all processes appeared to be flowing in an orderly fashion.

Soon Doctor Wayne needed some help; he waved toward me in my neutral corner and asked me to lend a hand. Before the night was over I had done more than just lend a hand. I learned to insert intravenous catheters, suture simple wounds, apply plaster casts and splints to arms and legs, and take blood pressures and vital signs. Being a part of some serious emergencies required me to dip into my limited store of knowledge and training and react before my brain or digestive system had time to register their own complaints. There was little time to know any patient. I compared the emergency department to the fast food drive-in experience of healthcare.

After a six hour blitz of patients the emergent activities quieted down in the early morning. Sometime during the evening the child with a bellyache had a large loose stool in his pants before he could make it to a toilet. This made his mom even more distraught. However, the abdominal pain resolved without surgery, and the mom literally dragged her child out of the emergency department yelling at him the entire way.

I learned to suture wounds on the three intoxicated men. To them I was just a young doctor. Nurse Murphy watched over my shoulder the entire time I was operating.

The impatient man who had double-parked his car in the tow away zone was attended after all the emergencies from the auto accidents had been cared for and appropriately discharged from the ER; some went home, some were admitted for observation, and some went to surgery.

Afterward Doctor Wayne sat me down and thanked me for my help. He told me that I was a pretty good hand and I could help him out any day. I thanked Dr. Wayne and Mrs. Murphy and told them I would return as much as I could. This would be my first of many visits to the emergency department to "learn and do" during my first two years in medical school.

After my first adventure in the ER I decided most doctors and nurses would agree that the emergency room was one place in the hospital they either loved or hated. I also learned that here the charge nurse was the controller, the mother, the protector, and the ultimate authority.

Early hospitals had what was called an emergency room because that area of the facility was used for one particular purpose only, emergencies. The ER was indeed just a single room. However, as the federal government became more involved in healthcare beginning in the 1950s, laws were passed making it illegal for any hospital or similar health related facility that received any form of federal compensation for healthcare services to deny access for emergencies to anyone. The penalty for denying services would be the forfeiture of all federal payments for healthcare services. The definition of an emergency was what *the patient* thought was an emergency and not what the healthcare providers thought. For the uninsured population or those who did not have a regular physician, the emergency room became the place to go when they were sick because it had to be open 24 hours a day and seven days a week. Over time emergency rooms became multi-roomed departments that were fully equipped with their own labs and CT scanners. The private physicians who used to cover the hospital emergency rooms could no longer keep up with the demand for their services most of which were not emergencies at all and new specialties in medicine and nursing were developed to staff the emergency departments.

Despite recent trends and governmental appeals for people to find their own family physicians, the use of hospital emergency departments for non-emergent primary care continues to increase. An article in the Journal of the American Medical Association in 2010 reported more than one hundred twenty million emergency department visits recorded. By 2014, the reported number of emergency department visits had increased to one hundred thirty-six million. After the Affordable Care Act, also known as Obamacare was instituted, the number of visits to a majority of hospitals' emergency departments increased by as much as twenty percent.[11,12,13]

The Medical School ER Nurse
Anonymous

Chief of Staff

Leaps tall buildings in a single bound
Is more powerful than a locomotive
Is faster than a speeding bullet
Walks on Water
Gives policy to God

Staff Doctor

Leaps short buildings in a single bound
Is more powerful than a switch engine
Is just as fast as a speeding bullet
Walks on water if the sea is calm
Talks with God

Resident

Leaps short buildings with a running bound
    and favorable winds
Is almost as powerful as a switch engine
Is faster than a speeding BB
Walks on water in a swimming pool
Talks with God if special request is approved

Intern

Clears a small hut
Loses a race with a locomotive
Can fire a speeding bullet
Swims well
Is occasionally addressed by God

Medical Student

Runs into small buildings
Recognized locomotive 2 out of 3 times
Wets himself with a water pistol
Dog paddles
Mumbles to animals

The Nurse

Lifts buildings to walk under
Kicks locomotives off the tracks
Catches speeding bullets in her teeth
Freezes water at a single glance
"She is God" ...

A Wake-up Call

In 1960, Cassius Clay, who would later to be called Muhammad Ali, became a professional boxer after winning the gold medal in the Olympics. The United States launched the world's first nuclear powered aircraft carrier named the USS Enterprise. The Soviet Union shot down an American U2 spy plane with pilot Frances Gary Powers aboard escalating cold war tensions. Computers were the size of small buildings and required their own refrigeration systems to control the heat they produced. The United States sent its first ground troops to Vietnam. A senator from Massachusetts named John Fitzgerald Kennedy became the youngest elected President of the United States. The laser and the first heart pacemaker were invented.[1]

During the summer of 1960, before I started the seventh grade, I was a diminutive thirteen-year-old boy who had no chance whatsoever of making any of the varsity athletic teams. At the encouragement of the football coach who made all the enrollment arrangements for me, I took a course in athletic training so I could become the athletic trainer for the junior high school sports teams. I learned to tape, bandage, splint, ice, and wrap all kinds of injuries. During this time I decided that I wanted to be a doctor someday, and this desire would never leave.

As a college undergraduate student at Eastern Montana College attempting to gain admission to medical school, I studied the sciences aggressively and eventually graduated with a degree in biology with an emphasis on population dynamics. Along the way, I worked as a teaching assistant in both biology and physics. Both disciplines taught me that the world must always maintain balance. For every up there must be a down; for every positive there must be negative; when a chemical reaction starts, then at some point it must stop. Along the way there are always winners and losers. That is nature's way.

My population biology background reminds me that living organisms, particularly microscopic ones that were the first living things, have taken over three hundred million years to evolve and find their unique places on this planet. As a rule, every species of organism had to meet the challenges of the day and find a place to survive or perish, or become extinct if you will. Alternatively, our so-called modern human experience is only about three hundred thousand years old, and human civilizations have existed for only about eight thousand years. Our biologic world is incomprehensibly complex, yet we humans keep trying to find simplistic solutions to keep all of our world's interwoven systems in balance.

One of my population biology classes was a study group in which all students and professors were expected to participate and to give input. The responsibility for developing questions for a session belonged to one of the professors, and each of the participants had their allotted time to give an answer to the questions of the day that had to exclude the human population.

One question was: "What would be the results upon various populations if a major predator were removed from an ecosystem?"

1. One the students in the group who was an avid hunter promptly stated that there would be more elk and deer for him to kill during hunting season.

2. Following up on this response, a botany professor interjected that there indeed would be more wild game, but they would eat more foliage. This could damage the plant ecosystem holding the soil together causing flooding if circumstances were appropriate.

3. Another professor who taught classes on bird watching promptly noted that with no trees and foliage, there would be no songbirds. Without songbirds, the bird predators such as eagles, crows, and hawks would move to where there was more food.

This type of discussion would continue for about thirty minutes or until everyone in the group had made a contribution.

Hunters carried out this very scenario in Yellowstone National Park and western Montana when wolves were essentially eliminated from the biologic system between 1900 and 1926. Within a few years the park rangers reported that the elk and deer herds were larger but did not appear to be as healthy because predators were not killing off the sickly ones. Additionally the larger numbers of animals overgrazed the meadows and all the smaller animals and birds that depended upon the grasses and small foliage started to disappear. Certainly the wolves had taken their toll on the farm and ranch animals in the past when they were present. In retrospect, however, the absence of wolves produced a much greater biologic disaster. Perhaps five years after the wolves were reintroduced into Yellowstone Park in 1995 after a seventy-year absence, the ecosystem had normalized. Nature rebalanced.[2,3]

Another question was: "What would we expect to happen to the aquatic populations if a dam were placed across a river?" The responses included:

1. In time, without the ability to migrate to spawn, a fish species would either have to adapt, or become extinct.
2. All the plant life that required a free flow of water would also have to adapt or die.
3. All of the larger animals that used the free flowing river for food may have to find another location for food.
4. All the microbes or bacteria that resided in the aquatic organisms or in the water also would have to adapt or perish.

Again the central theme of the discussions was that nature would eventually become balanced by adaptation of the species. Actually this scenario took place naturally in August 1959, in mountainous southwestern Montana when a massive earthquake produced landslides and created a new lake named Quake Lake.[4] This phenomenon of adaptation also occurs each time a permanent dam is constructed to control flooding and to produce hydroelectric power, or when a hurricane blows through the landscape, or when a new germ like the AIDS virus comes along. The biologic system will adapt in time.

I mention these instances to reinforce the concept that Mother Nature always wins. She makes the corrections on her time, not human time. Again one must remember that for every action there must be an equal and opposite reaction to keep the natural world in balance. When changes occur or are man-made, the law of unintended consequences often prevails. All too often the remedy for a perceived problem is worse than the illness. What humans think is a long time to correct a concern, perhaps a century or sometimes even as little as a week, natural forces may take thousands or even millions of years to correct. The natural system always adapts eventually. This is the way it has always been for millennia.

I refer to these episodes along with the corresponding thought processes used by population biologists like me because my going to medical school became an adventure into a foreign land. Doctors did not worry about, nor were medical students taught about, global biology issues when they were trying to treat or cure patients. Not once did I hear a professor share any concern about the consequences of using antibiotics. Even infectious disease specialists who spent their entire lives obliterating germs, or trying to obliterate them, never seemed to concern themselves with what may be happening to the rest of their patient's millions or more species of *normal* germs killed by broad spectrum antibiotics. The idea I guess was similar to dropping atomic bombs in Japan when nobody knew exactly what was going to happen; they would just have to wait and see. I learned surgical phrases such as, "When in doubt, cut it out." My favorite quote was when a staff physician was talking with a lab technician about a bacteria culture report. The lab technician reported the result was normal flora. The doctor yelled out loudly, "I don't care what flora it is! I just want to know what will kill the damn things!" Obviously if the bacteria were all normal, then nothing needed to be killed with antibiotics. Shortsighted thinking like this always bothered me.

The past, current and potential long-term costs of this type of thinking regarding the organisms that we cannot see or know much about is well delineated in *Missing Microbes,* a 2014 book written by Martin Blaser M.D.[5]

When my medical school class was nearing graduation, Dr. Robert Bacon, the admissions committee chairman, reaffirmed what he had told us early on in our four-year journey to become doctors, "Remember that half of what you have learned will be false in five years. We just don't know which half, so keep on learning." Another advisor who was a physician in private practice told me, "Don't believe anything you hear and only half of what you see. Be curious. Keep looking for not only *an* answer but for the *correct* answer." Our advisors taught us how to conduct ourselves when we engaged in the private practice of medicine. It did not dawn on me until sometime later that the professors who were giving us advice had never been in a private practice of medicine. As it turned out, young doctors were pretty much on their own when it came to establishing a private medical practice. Corporations employed few doctors in the 1970s like they do in the 21st century.

Setting up a private medical practice required a steep learning curve. Not only was I expected to practice up-to-date medicine, but also my personal expectation was to keep current in scientific thought as best as humanly possible. Additionally, as a young physician I had to learn about the politics of medicine and hospital care, the financing of healthcare, and the expectations of the community for activities outside the realm of medicine. I enjoyed the challenges of a medical practice in a rural area of Montana. After the initial culture shock of becoming a new physician, I soon knew that my calling to medicine was the correct one.

Over the past half century I saw and experienced many changes in medicine and healthcare. Whether the changes are considered good or bad will require much more time. We are all on the same road going to one final destination, but each individual's journey is unique. I have come to appreciate that no two people have the same story, not even twins. I have had the good fortune of being able to provide care for a broad spectrum of patients including newborn infants struggling to inhale their first breaths to senior citizens who had lived a century or more and many others in between who have allowed me to help them along their many special journeys through life.

The Kids' Surgeon

Graduating from medical school in 1974 was a momentary highlight after my four years of intense academic effort. Just like graduating from high school and from college, the euphoria was short-lived since I would be moving on with my wife Kay and baby Jennifer to another adventure, a rotating internship. After graduating with a Doctor of Medicine degree on a Saturday afternoon in June, Kay and I packed up our few possessions, loaded them into a U-Haul trailer during the weekend, and drove to Spokane, Washington, where I was to start my internship the following week.

It just so happened that the World's Fair was in Spokane that summer and housing for new interns was scarce. The Sacred Heart Hospital where I would be training did have a room for each intern if the new doctor decided to stay at the hospital full-time. Unfortunately, these accommodations certainly were not appropriate for families. After several days of searching Kay and I found an acceptable rental home in northeast Spokane about five miles from the hospital. I purchased a new bicycle so that I could commute the distance and save money. At the time interns received only $550 per month plus meals at the hospital.

My graduating medical school class was the last to be required to take a rotating internship. These training programs were also called Iron Man Internships because of the amount of time and effort required to complete the year of training. Indeed, not too many years before me, the young doctors lived in the hospital for the entire duration of their training. Medical training hour rules were changed the next year after I graduated and newly graduated medical students had to choose a course of further study after medical school, such as surgery, psychiatry, or pediatrics. I had always wanted to be a generalist family doctor in a rural community, like the physicians in the television program *Marcus Welby, MD*

After several days of intern orientation and taking classes to become certified in adult and pediatric cardiopulmonary resuscitation, critical care protocols, and trauma patient evaluation, each intern was given a schedule of medical discipline rotations for the coming year. All interns had to complete thirteen four-week rotations that included pediatrics, general surgery, obstetrics, emergency room, orthopedics, surgical intensive care, cardiac intensive care, general medicine, and four weeks of elective rotations. My program started with two four-week rotations in pediatrics.

The pediatricians in private practice each had assigned periods of time when they served as preceptors for interns on the hospital's pediatric service. During the first few days of my pediatric rotation, I had the opportunity to meet with all the pediatricians. Each doctor arrived in the hospital dressed with a suit and tie and each told us his expectations of what he expected the interns to do for him in return for his supervision.

Midday on the Friday afternoon of my first week in pediatrics I was summoned to the nurses' station by the head nurse. She advised me that Dr. Chadwick Baxter, the hospital's pediatric surgeon, wanted to meet me and that he would be on the pediatrics floor soon, and the nurse asked me to wait at the nurses' station for him. I had waited no more than a few minutes when I saw a man coming down the hallway who looked more like a farmer than a doctor. The man was short of stature but powerfully built from the waist up. He had an obvious saddle deformity of his nose and thinning gray hair. He wore faded jeans, a long-sleeved flannel shirt with the sleeves rolled up to the mid forearm, and a string bolo tie. On his hip connected to his belt was a large Motorola radio. Dr. Baxter certainly did not look like the other pediatricians that I had met.

When he arrived at the nurses' station, I introduced myself. He in turn identified himself as Chad Baxter, the local kids' surgeon. He explained that his job was to teach me a few things about surgery. He knew what the other pediatricians wanted me

to do for them and their patients; however, he related that he
wanted nothing from me except my attention. He then informed
me that during my eight-week pediatrics rotation he would be
my preceptor for seven consecutive days. He was quite emphatic
that during those seven days I belonged to him, and him alone.
He also told me that any other time that he was doing surgery,
and I was free from my other duties, I was more than welcome to
assist him with the operations. After a few more pleasantries, he
told me it was Friday afternoon and he was off to his farm.

One day when I was on call I had the opportunity to assist
Dr. Baxter with an emergency procedure on a child late in the
evening. Dr. Baxter asked if I wanted to watch or if I wanted to
assist him with the operation. Promptly I told him I would like
to assist. At that point he took me aside, picked up a needle
holder and a needle with suture, and asked me to show him if I
could put a stitch into a towel and tie a surgical knot with the
suture.

Without hesitation I picked up the needle holder, inserted the
needle, and proceeded to put stitches into the towel. After I
placed two stitches in the towel, Dr. Baxter asked me where I
learned to grip the needle holder. I informed him that I learned
how to hold the instruments at the Veterans Hospital at the University of Oregon Medical School, and the surgeon's name was
Dr. Phillip Snedeker.

Dr. Baxter then told me that I was the first intern in ten
years to know how to hold a needle driver correctly and that Dr.
Snedeker had taught me well. Dr. Baxter then invited me to
assist him with his surgery to show him what else I knew. I
believe he wanted to make sure I was not going to be an impedi-
ment to him or the surgical team during the operation. I figured
that when he asked me to scrub my hands and get ready I had
passed his first test. Before this surgical case started Dr. Baxter
asked me what the four most important things were in doing
surgery on children. I confessed I did not know.

He followed with:
1   be gentle,
2   be gentle,
3   Be Gentle,
4   and, by the way, always BE GENTLE!

He smiled and asked, "Any questions?"

I nodded that I understood.

I had the chance to be in the operating room with Dr. Baxter on several more occasions before my week with him officially arrived. Fortunately, I had not made any major mistakes, as far as he would tell me anyway. My week with Dr. Baxter arrived, and the days were pretty much twenty-four hours on call followed by twenty-four more hours on call. Dr. Baxter was the only pediatric surgeon within three hundred miles or more, and he was very particular about who took care of his patients and never asked me or any other intern to do so. He said there was enough stress in just learning about children with surgery. It was his job to assume the stress while the interns could relax and learn.

One afternoon after I had already completed my week, Dr. Baxter asked me to come to the emergency room if I had time. He had an eleven-year-old female patient who had been referred by her family doctor from a small town some distance away. A young girl, who was accompanied by her mother, was complaining of severe pain in her right lower abdomen. On examination, Dr. Baxter showed me a mass in that area. Hernias in females are rare, but it appeared to me this child had one in her lower abdomen on the right side with something stuck in it. Most likely, I assumed, it would be a piece of intestine. At any rate, the child was quite ill with persistent nausea and vomiting, and it was obvious that she was going to require an operation to repair the problem.

After the appropriate testing had been ordered and the consents for surgery had been signed, Dr. Baxter and I walked toward the locker rooms to don scrub suits. Within a short time we joined the young girl in the operating room where the doctor reassured her about what he was going to do and that everything was going to be okay. He told her that when she woke up her mother would be in the room with her.

The anesthetist put the child to sleep and her abdomen was prepared for the operation. Dr. Baxter assumed his usual position on the right side of the patient while I settled in on the left side to be his assistant. At that point he looked at me and said, "Dr. Ashcraft, we've already fixed hernias together. I think its time for you to do one by yourself." He then invited me to change places with him at the operating table. This was something that surgeons usually did not do with the interns. I felt honored.

As I started the operation, making sure to be gentle, I opened the tissues above the mass. Immediately in front of me I had exposed this young girl's ovary. Adjacent to her ovary was the end of her fallopian tube that appeared to have a bulge approximately half an inch from the end. I had no idea what I was dealing with. After a short discussion, Dr. Baxter reassured me that I could complete the operation. He tapped my gloved hand with his index finger and told me he was not going anywhere. This made me feel better but not any less anxious.

Now Dr. Baxter asked the surgical nurse to obtain a catheterized urine specimen from the youngster and to perform a pregnancy test.

The nurse responded that the child was only eleven years old.

Dr. Baxter assured the nurse that he was aware of the child's age, but he was just covering all bases. He asked another nurse to have the pathologist oversee the test and call the results to the operating room. Obviously sensing potential legal issues, Dr. Baxter also asked the nurse supervisor to have two other people validate that the urine sample came from this child.

After the nurse obtained a urine sample, oversaw the appropriate signatures, and sent the sample to the lab, I continued with my delicate dissection in this area. Needless to say I was extremely nervous but Dr. Baxter was patient and kept whispering for me to take my time and be gentle.

Within a few minutes a voice came over the loudspeaker in the operating room. The voice rang out, "Chad, the pregnancy test is positive. Do you want me to do anything else?"

Dr. Baxter asked the pathologist not to leave until he had a chance to evaluate the initial surgical specimen. The pathologist replied that he would stay in the lab until further notice.

After I had all the tissues separated and easily identifiable, Dr. Baxter asked me what I was going to do next. I told him that I thought the child had an ectopic pregnancy in her fallopian tube and guessed I would have to remove all the involved tissues. Before we did anything, Dr. Baxter asked the surgical nurse to bring in a camera so that we could take pictures of our specimens and the operative site.

Dr. Baxter replied, "That's what I would expect a general surgeon or a gynecologist to do." However, this was a child, and he was not going to jeopardize the rest of her reproductive life by doing something rash. Therefore, he suggested that we remove the small ectopic pregnancy and suture the fallopian tube back together. I knew that performing this procedure was way out of my league in terms of the operative skill required. However, instead of just taking over the case, Dr. Baxter asked me if I would allow him to show me what he thought we should do.

I promptly agreed.

At this point Dr. Baxter asked for some magnifying spectacles, and after putting them on, he meticulously and extremely carefully opened the fallopian tube, shelled out the ectopic pregnancy and sent it to pathology. He then closed the fallopian tube with tiny sutures used by the ophthalmologists when they worked on the eyeball.

When he was done, Dr. Baxter thanked me for allowing him to assist and then asked me to finish the operation. At this point I was able to reinsert the ovary and the repaired fallopian tube back into the abdomen and then close the hernia defect in the abdominal wall. When I finished closing the skin wound Dr. Baxter thanked me again for allowing him to assist with the operation.

Before we left the operating room, Dr. Baxter asked the nurse assistants to draw up the child's legs so that more pictures could be obtained of the child's genital area. On preliminary evaluation it appeared to me that she had received substantial trauma around her genital area, and more than likely she had been raped.

Back in the locker room while we were getting dressed Dr. Baxter asked me if I knew what we had just seen. Before I could reply, he told me that the chance of having a female with a hernia is about one percent. The chance of that hernia having an ovary is about one in a thousand. And the chance of that fallopian tube having an ectopic pregnancy in an eleven-year-old child is astronomical. Therefore, we had just seen and repaired something that was not only rare but also extraordinarily rare, perhaps one in ten million or more.

I told Dr. Baxter that I was glad he was there and I appreciated the learning experience. He thanked me for helping. He told me that he had never seen or heard of a similar case and thought he might report it in a journal.

Before we left the locker room Dr. Baxter told me that if anyone asked, he did all the surgery. He advised me that there were going to be some legal issues and police involved with this case, and it was his job to be the point man. He thanked me for my efforts and told me again I did a good job.

When I made my way back to the pediatric ward I could see Dr. Baxter in the hallway talking with the mother, two men in suits, and some police officers. They obviously had many social and legal issues that needed to be resolved; I was glad I only had to help repair the girl's surgical problem. I never learned who raped her.

It just so happened that Doctor Baxter was extremely busy with emergencies the week I was with him. Along with my other duties in the hospital for being on call and taking emergencies for the pediatric floor every other day, I did not leave the hospital premises for nine consecutive days. That means that I was working or available for duty in the hospital for over two hundred consecutive hours. I would later learn that when I was on the surgery service those eighteen-hour days, seven days a week were the normal working hours for interns, at least for me. I was so busy I felt as if I carried a black cloud over my head. Years later our local surgeon called me Joe Btfsplk, the character in the *L'il Abner* cartoons who carried the same image over his head. The interns following me in the years to come could expect a far less rigorous training experience brought on by government regulations that changed training mandates. I was convinced the new training programs would not be as good or as beneficial as the one I was having. As a future instructor in medicine I would find out first hand how the modified training rules had diminished the overall medical training experience.

About ten years later physician training in the United States took a drastic and unexpected turn. An eighteen-year-old woman named Libby Zion went to the emergency room of the New York Hospital, now the New York Presbyterian Cornell Medical Center, on March 4, 1984, and died unexpectedly less than twenty-four hours later from a rare drug interaction that was unknown at the time. She had been seen, evaluated, and treated by resident doctors in the hospital. The circumstances of her death prompted her father, who was an influential publisher, to have murder charges filed against the treating doctors in the hospital. The doctors and the hospital were absolved of criminal negligence some years later. Nevertheless, a New York state commission named the Bell Commission subsequently recommended in 1989 sweeping changes in the ways that doctors were trained and supervised in New York State hospitals and medical schools. Soon thereafter these changes regarding faculty supervisory responsibilities and allowable working hours for residents and interns became nationwide standards and transformed the way doctors could be trained. Looking back on the experience I had with Dr. Baxter during that week of more than hundred twenty hours, I knew that the young doctors of today could not possibly have the same learning experience by working a mandatory maximum eighty-hour week.[14,15]

About five years after my internship when I was in private practice a young female patient come to our emergency department with a similar problem of a mass in the lower abdomen associated with pain. She too had something stuck in an abdominal wall hernia. As I was about to make a skin incision to start the operation I remembered Dr. Baxter's admonition for surgery in children, "Be gentle!" On this occasion the offending object in the hernia defect was a normal appendix that had become stuck. This time the procedure and the circumstances were much simpler, but I knew what to do.

The chance of a female having an inguinal hernia, a hole in the lower abdominal wall, is approximately one percent. The chance of an appendix being in the hernia defect is about one in a thousand cases. Once again, I encountered a rare surgical condition.

A few years later I was the program coordinator for the Montana Academy of Family Physicians. I was fortunate to recruit Dr. Baxter to speak about surgical care of the child and outpatient surgical procedures. He was indeed a hit with the record number of attendees at the meeting. After his prepared remarks, which lasted an hour, Dr. Baxter continued with an impromptu question and answer session for an additional two hours. He would have continued but I had to interrupt him so the evening session could start on time.

As Dr. Baxter was preparing to leave the conference and return to Spokane, I reminded him of the case of the pregnant child when I was an intern, which he remembered, and I reported to him the case I had in my private practice several years before.

First, he thanked me for allowing him the opportunity to be a guest speaker at the conference and to get away from Spokane and his busy practice. Next, Dr. Baxter apologized for not being able to talk about everything that I had asked him to cover in his program. And finally, with a smile he inquired about my surgical procedure, "Were you gentle?"

"Yes, I was," I replied and smiled.

Rubbed the Wrong Way

Despite promises from the city fathers that we would have suitable housing when we arrived in Sidney, Montana, none was available. The excuse was that the town was in the middle of an oil boom and housing was a premium commodity. After finding no acceptable housing, Kay and our daughter Jennifer moved to Bozeman, Montana, to live with her parents while I spent the first month of my time in Sidney sleeping on a basement floor in a sleeping bag. During the next month, Kay and I negotiated to buy a new home from a banker and his wife who had received an immediate job transfer and needed to sell their newly built home promptly. In the middle part of June 1976 my family and I moved into a six-month-old home located on ten acres five miles north of Sidney.

Soon after our telephone service was installed, we started to receive calls that weren't for us. Our phone connection had been set up as a country party line, and we received all of our neighbors' phone calls, day and night. Additionally, all the neighbors were listening each time a phone call was made to us. Initially, the people at the phone company told us that we couldn't have a private line in our neighborhood and the best they would offer us was a two-party line. The rationale was that only two people would be aware of what patients were talking about when they called me. Kay and I both told them that that situation was not acceptable, and we demanded to have a single party line to our home because of my job or we would find an alternative. We then started to investigate the possibility of having a two-way radio system for communication.

Not long after this discussion with the local phone company we received a phone call from the regional office of the phone company notifying us that they had installed a private line to our home. The company made sure to remind us that our phone line was the only private line in our neighborhood.

The new private line worked well for about two weeks until very early on a Saturday morning loud pounding on our front door awakened us. As I approached the front door I could see a flashing light in our driveway. When I opened the front door a large deputy sheriff confronted me and asked if I was Dr. Ashcraft. After I confirmed my name, the officer told me that the hospital had been trying to contact me by phone and they needed me at the hospital immediately to deliver a baby. I thanked the officer for contacting me and told him I would get to the hospital as soon as I could. I then listened on our phone receiver and heard nothing but static.

Kay wanted to know what was going on. I relayed the deputy sheriff's comments, I told her the phones weren't working and that I would return from the hospital when I was done. She wanted to know why the hospital had called me because I was not the doctor on call.

I had no idea.

As I was driving to town in the middle of the night I thought to myself that I had been in Sidney only about two months, I knew I had no obstetric patients waiting to deliver, and I wondered why the hospital sent the sheriff out to my home when four other doctors, who lived right in town and only short distances from the hospital, could have easily responded to the emergency. In particular, there was a specific doctor on call for emergencies at the hospital.

The ER nurse met me at the door leading to the doctor's parking lot and encouraged me to hurry to the delivery room because a woman was about to have her baby. She gave me no further details. When I arrived in the delivery room suite I could see a young pregnant woman on the delivery table crying with pain along with a nurse's aide at her side who was holding her hand and keeping a cool wash cloth on the her forehead. Before I changed my clothes, I examined the woman, learned from her that this was her first baby, and determined that she probably had at least another hour of labor before she had a baby. I tried to reassure the nurse and the patient that all was going well and that I would return as soon as I put on surgical attire. Within a few minutes I returned to the obstetric suite to attend this woman's delivery. While we were waiting I learned that not only was this my new patient's first pregnancy but also it was the first delivery for the nurse and the nursing aide.

Eventually the young woman had a natural birth of a vigorous female infant. Instead of exultation at the birth of a baby, the three women in the room seemed exhausted and relieved that the ordeal was over. When I alerted the nurse to have family members come into the delivery room to see the new baby, if the mother wished, the nurse whispered into my ear that the woman was having the baby out of wedlock and that no family members were in the hospital. I then put the baby onto the mother's chest for the two to have some bonding time while I examined and repaired the woman's external genital area.

After I assured myself that the mother and baby were doing well and both had been transferred out of the delivery room suite, I dictated a delivery note. Afterward I asked the nurse why she did not call the doctor on ER call or one of the other doctors in town since they were so much closer. She informed me that none of the doctors, even the one on call, would not come to see the woman in labor because each knew the family and were convinced they wouldn't be paid. For whatever reason the doctors just didn't want to get involved in the middle of the night.

The nurse then told me that when she called my home she got a recorded message saying, "Not in service." Therefore, since she assumed I was home, the nurse dispatched the County Sheriff to get me. Before I left the hospital I first called my home to verify its dysfunction and then the telephone company to advise them of my dilemma.

The next day a repairman came to our home to fix our non-functioning telephone. After an hour or so the repairman asked me to accompany him into my field. He and I walked about two hundred yards south across my field to my neighbor's fence, which was the boundary line between our two properties. The man showed me a plastic coated wire that had been secured to one of the fence posts with staples and told me that this was my private phone line laying across the barbed wire fence. The repairman showed me where the cable had been laid down in the irrigation drainage ditches on both properties and then pointed further south toward several cows that were grazing in a pasture. He told me, "Cows like nothing better than to rub against fence posts." Pointing again at the wire secured to the fencepost, the man showed me where the staples had worn through the plastic coating after a lot of friction from rubbing and the phone signal was shorting out on the barbed wire fence. Somewhat disgusted, the repairman commented that sometimes people, even those working for the phone company, took shortcuts during the oil boom. He admitted that our phone line connection was definitely a shortcut.

The repairman removed the damaged section of cable and spliced in a section of new wire to allow our phone to work temporarily. He told me the appropriate repair would require a new trench from the junction box that was located further south down the road from my neighbor's land to our home. Because of the backlog of work at the phone company, he could not guess when that work would be completed. Before finishing, the man put a protective cap over the wire where it was attached to the fence post to keep the cows from damaging it again.

The trencher team came about a week later, installed our private phone line, and removed the wire cable from the neighbor's fence and irrigation ditches. We had no further party-line problems with our phone service for the next twenty-five years.

I discussed the incident with the other doctors at a special medical staff meeting the next Tuesday. The established doctors essentially told me they would attend whatever patient they chose whether or not they were on call for the hospital. It was their choice, not the patient's or the hospital's. Several doctors commented that the town and the hospital should be glad they were available at all.

What could I say?

From that day forward my commitment to our new community was that whenever I was summoned to the hospital, I would go.

The cows continued to enjoy rubbing on my neighbor's fence posts, but it no longer bothered our telephone reception.

Martha

Sidney, Montana, was an oil boomtown in the late 1970s and early 1980s. The patient volume in our small rural hospital and our clinic was almost unbearable. Seldom was I putting in less than a sixteen-hour day. I was in our clinic late on a Friday afternoon and had been up caring for patients for almost twenty-four hours. The other physician with whom I worked had left town about a week before to visit his family in western Montana. Unfortunately, he became stranded in a wintry ice storm that kept him from returning to town to take his scheduled rotation for emergency calls. To be sure, I was not looking forward to another long weekend in the hospital awaiting more seriously ill and trauma patients in the emergency room. After I had seen my last clinic patient for the day and as I was dictating my medical records, my nurse Georgia came into my office to tell me that there was a woman on the telephone who wished to talk to me. Georgia gave me no further information.

As I lifted the phone receiver and introduced myself I heard a woman's voice ask, "Is this the doctor?"

I replied that I was indeed Dr. Ashcraft. I asked if there was something I could do to help her.

The woman informed me that she lived on an isolated farm in western North Dakota perhaps a ninety minutes to two hours drive away from Sidney. She wondered if I would mind if she asked me a medical question.

Certainly she could ask a question.

The woman introduced herself as Martha. She related that she had something curious happening with her body, and she wanted to know if it was serious or not.

I asked her to continue with her story.

Martha told me that she noted that her stools in the toilet were flat. She wondered if that was a problem.

I asked her what she meant by flat. I inquired if the stools were just smaller than usual or if they were actually flat like a pancake.

She replied that they were flat more like a thick ribbon, and she had noticed this phenomenon for about six months.

When I asked if the stools had changed color or if she had appreciated anything looking like blood in the toilet, she said no.

I then asked Martha multiple questions that doctors often use when they are trying to get more information about a change in stool patterns. For each question Martha gave a negative response.

After this short discussion, I advised Martha that it would be best if I could see her in person to perform a physical examination and evaluate her more fully. I told her that since she had been having symptoms for over six months I did not believe she had an emergency to deal with. I requested that she come to see me in the clinic the upcoming Monday.

Martha answered that would be fine except it would have to be in the afternoon, perhaps late in the day. She noted that there was considerable snow and ice on the country roads, and she had farm chores to perform as well as to make sure that her family and workers were fed.

I assured her that I would see her when she arrived in Sidney no matter what the hour. She agreed to an appointment, gave me her home number, and hung up the phone. I called in my nurse to place a note on Monday's appointment book to make sure that I did not miss my appointment with Martha, whenever it was.

Over the weekend the wintry weather worsened. For a short time no highway traffic was advised in or out of town. However, the bad weather did not prevent the continuous stream of patients with their oilfield related accidents into our emergency room. Consequently, I did not leave the hospital to go home the entire weekend. When Monday morning came I was supposed to be off the call schedule. Unfortunately, Dr. Smythe was still isolated in western Montana because of the bad weather. I resolved to being available for emergency calls until he returned.

Martha came into the clinic a little after lunch. Since I was seeing patients in the hospital at the time, Georgia paged me to inform me of Martha's arrival. In a few minutes I was in my clinic ready for my new patient who my nurse had already seated in an examination room. Upon entering I viewed a middle-aged woman who was meticulously groomed and dressed as if she were going out to attend an important event. The woman stood up, I introduced myself and extended my right hand to shake hers, and after we had shaken hands we both sat down.

Before I started to ask about Martha's medical concerns, I asked her a few personal questions about herself and her family. Martha informed me that she was now sixty-two years old. She and her husband had married just after they graduated from high school. Together, they had five children, three sons and two daughters. The daughters were grown-up, college-educated, married, had several children each, and had moved with their families out of state. The three sons had all finished college. Two of the men remained on the ranch and were married with children while one son was working out of state as an engineer. Her husband had died from a heart attack while working on the ranch several years before.

I then asked Martha to tell me about her health problems. She told me that for about six months she thought her stools appeared to be flat like a ribbon. She told me that she did not feel bad, her appetite was good, she did not feel sick, she had not lost any weight, and she seemed to have as much energy as ever. Yet, she stated that it just didn't seem right for her stools to change like that. When I asked if she had noticed any blood in the toilet or on the stool itself she replied that she had not noticed any blood or black stools.

At this point Martha said, "I've got something to show you." She then reached into a bag and pulled out yet other plastic bag that contained a cottage cheese container. Inside this container was a sample of her stool that she had obtained for me just that morning. Indeed, the stool was about a quarter inch thick and flat just as she had described. I took a piece of the stool out of the container with a tongue depressor and placed the sample on a blood-testing card that was available in all of my examination rooms. (This is termed testing for occult blood and the name of the card is Hemoccult.) When I applied the testing solution to the sample, the card instantly turned blue indicating that there was a significant amount of blood in the sample. I knew immediately from Martha's history of a flat stool and now blood in the stool that she had a cancer in her colon. I also suspected that since she had been noticing the flat stools for six months or better, the cancer was more than likely widely spread which made her prognosis grim.

I asked Martha to disrobe and put on an examination gown after I stepped out of the room. After a few moments I returned to perform a physical examination. My examination was essentially normal except that I could feel a mass at the tip of my finger as I performed a rectal examination. Interestingly, I was unable to appreciate any mass in Martha's thin lower abdomen when I examined her a second time. After Martha dressed, we had an opportunity to discuss my findings. I explained to her that I felt a mass in her bowel and that along with the blood in her stool certainly concerned me and warranted further investigation.

Martha wanted to know if she had cancer. I could only say that I did not know for sure. Technically this was true because a final diagnosis could only be made after biopsy had been obtained, but I was almost positive that she had an advanced colon cancer. After another short discussion, Martha agreed to begin testing in the hospital that afternoon; I had Georgia make the necessary arrangements.

After the bowel was cleaned out following several days of water enemas to remove all remnants of stool, I performed a sigmoidoscopy whereby a lighted tube is inserted into the rectum to look for abnormalities. After being inserted only a short distance the instrument encountered an obstruction in the bowel that looked a large piece of cauliflower. I could not find an opening in the intestine with this test.

Subsequently, I asked the radiologist to perform X-rays with a contrasting dye called a barium enema. Before the days of CT scanning, which became commonplace in the early 1980s and MRIs, which came a few year's later, we used an x-ray test called a barium enema whereby a dilute contrast material was inserted into the bowel while standard x-rays were performed. These pictures gave us some idea of what was inside the bowel.

Afterward the radiologist called me into his office to review the pictures. He showed me an x-ray with a lesion that appeared like a partially eaten apple core lesion in Martha's lower colon that was a classic picture for a large cancer. The radiologist showed me where the tumor was almost totally obstructing the bowel. He also pointed out several dark irregular spots in the pelvic bones where the bone was missing. To him these lesions appeared very much like metastatic cancer.

Soon after the x-rays were obtained, I talked with Martha about our findings. She did not seem to be very upset by my report. She did note that her children should see the results and hear what I had to say in person because she did not want to get anything mixed up. Thereafter, Martha said she would arrange for her family to come into town with her the next morning to discuss the findings. In the meantime, I had discussions with the hospital pathologist and our local surgeon to review Martha's case. The pathologist taught me that if the lesions in the bone were actually metastatic disease then my patient's days were numbered. Statistically, the doctor thought my patient *might* have three to six months to live unless, he cautioned, "The oncologists didn't get to her." The surgeon agreed to see Martha after the family conference adjourned the next day.

The family meeting occurred the next morning as planned. With all members present I reviewed the x-ray films and reports that were completed, reviewed the laboratory tests that were done, and told them that I had already discussed the situation with the local doctors. Martha and her children all agreed that she should have a surgery to remove the tumor if for no other reason than to prevent a total bowel obstruction, a situation that

would require an emergency operation. Even though Martha
had no medical insurance, the family members assured her that
they would find a way to pay the bills. Martha insisted that she
would not have a colostomy, a surgical opening of the large intestine onto the abdominal wall that is connected to a bag that col-
lects stool.

Several days later Martha underwent surgery to remove the
colon tumor during which the surgeon, the pathologist, and I
determined the mass was cancerous and had spread, or metasta-
sized, to other places in her abdomen. The surgeon wanted to
remove more bowel tissue and make a colostomy, but I reminded
him of Martha's wishes. Therefore, a colostomy was not made
and the woman's rectum was preserved even though we knew
that the area might still have cancerous tissue.

During her postoperative recovery Martha and I had the
opportunity to talk about her prognosis. She wanted to know how
long she had to live. Truthfully, I told her I had no idea; I could
give her statistics based on averages, but knowing exactly how
long she would live was what I always called a God question
because only He knew the answer.

After the surgery, the surgeon arranged for Martha to be seen
by a cancer care specialist, or oncologist, in Billings, Montana, to
discuss the possibility of further cancer treatment with
chemotherapy or radiation. The surgeon told Martha that he
thought the chemotherapy should start in about six weeks when
her wounds were well healed.

Martha was reluctant to take any more treatments because, as
she told me, she would just be a bother to her family, and she did
not have enough money to pay the bills. Yet, after talking with her
family members, all of whom wanted her to take more treatments,
Martha kept the appointment with the oncology doctor.

About eight weeks later Martha came into my clinic unan-
nounced and without an appointment. Georgia, knowing that I
would need a considerable amount of time to counsel her, had
Martha return toward the end of the day so we would not be

bothered. Martha and I met after I'd seen my last scheduled patient in the clinic.

As usual Martha came to the clinic immaculately dressed. No one would know anything was medically wrong by her appearance alone. She wanted to talk with me about her visit and discussions with the oncologist and his team. Martha told me that she had not discussed anything about that visit with her family. Martha pointedly told me that she wanted me to answer the God question. That is, how long was she going to live and be comfortable? She wanted to know how much the chemotherapy was going to make her suffer because that seemed to be something the oncologist and his team did not want to approach, and, according to Martha, the oncologist seemed to get upset when she even questioned his course of treatment. The cost of the entire process was most important to her, and the cancer specialists dodged the discussion entirely. Finally, Martha wanted to know how much longer she could expect to live if she took the chemotherapy treatments and survived.

My initial response was another question, "What exactly did the oncologist tell you?"

Martha reached into her purse and pulled out a piece of paper with some writing on it. Martha told me that she wrote down exactly what the doctor said just before he insisted that she should start chemotherapy right away. She handed me the note that read:

"There is a reasonable probability that there is a very good possibility that we might be able to help you live longer."

When I read the statement all I could think of was, "What a bunch of double talk!"

When I asked Martha what she thought about the statement, she said that initially all she heard were the words "help you live longer." She wrote down the doctor's statement so that everyone in her family understood what was said. Afterward, when she looked at the statement again, Martha told me she had no idea what it meant.

I told Martha that to me the statement was gobbledygook. I informed her that with a cancer that was as widely spread in the body as hers, she would be quite fortunate to live another year. The chemotherapy treatments, if they worked, might give her at most a few more weeks or perhaps a few months to live. Unfortunately, in the meantime she would be miserable most of the time. My educated guess was the cost of treatment would be more than $150,000 without any complications.

Martha told me that being sick at the end of your life should not have to cost someone or their family their entire life's savings. She pointed out, and quite accurately, that the cancer doctors don't make a living if they can't prescribe poisons to sick people. She questioned me about the Hippocratic oath that says, "Do no harm." Finally, Martha told me that the native Indians cared for the sick and elderly in a much better way. She told me the sick and the elderly were just left behind when the tribe moved on, and they let Mother Nature take its course.

After we discussed a few more topics of concern to Martha, she asked about returning in a week or so to chat again. I assured her that I looked forward to our next visit.

When time allowed I telephoned the oncologist in Billings, Montana, who had attended Martha and who was well respected in Montana as a hematologist and oncologist. I was concerned about his comments to Martha that seemed to me to be less than forthright. Additionally, I was bothered about his skirting some of the issues that Martha raised. Essentially, he did not admit to anything unusual with the way he cared for Martha compared to his other cancer patients. He did acknowledge, however, that their group usually did not discuss financial concerns with patients because of the doctors' lack of financial expertise and because some patients might decline treatment because of the cost. He and his associates in the hematology department tended to be positive when it came to discussing longevity concerns.

I thought his answers avoided the issues with me too, and from that conversation forward I became much more wary of what the cancer doctors told my patients. Even though I referred many patients for cancer treatment over the next twenty-five years, I became much more cynical about the true value of such treatments. The way doctors, hospitals, and drug companies using mass media present cancer studies erroneously still bothers me today.

Doctors are trained to evaluate, diagnose, and take care of illness, and I suppose that during our training we learn to lean toward optimism when it comes to discussing cancer patients' long-term health or their prognoses for survival. Some doctors seem as if they know the answers to God questions, but they really don't. There are probably many reasons why doctors, especially those tending the very sick and dying, tend to be optimistic. I wonder if the emotional drain on patients with severe disease can be matched by the emotional drain on the doctors who care for the sickest patients day in and day out. Unfortunately, life expectancy prognostications do not have a scientific basis. Perhaps some doctors improve their own optimism and mental health by embellishing the facts pertaining to the life expectancy of their patients with life threatening diseases.

In 2000, one study from England pointed out that cancer specialists overestimated their patients remaining days by five hundred percent.[16] Another study posted in 2001[17] from America revealed that doctors' optimism appeared to be a deliberate, but hopefully well-intentioned, strategy to give dying patients hope. In this study as many as one-third of the nation's cancer specialists in the study intentionally overestimated their patients' life expectancies. Obviously, many doctors dealing with the very sick and dying try to find their own personal balance between science and compassion. Dr. Peter Ubel from Duke University pointed out, "The truth we communicate to patients should help them prepare for the worst while allowing them to hope for the best."[18]

Numerous articles have been written about miraculous cancer treatments enticing patients and doctors to use them. The fact is that so far patients are not getting much bang for their healthcare dollars, but pharmaceutical companies and cancer doctors are doing quite well financially with Americans spending more than $23 billion yearly for potential cancer cures. Despite claims to the contrary, history reminds us that rarely are cancers cured. Dr. David Howard from Emory University's Department of Health Policy and Management notes, "In general, the progress for cancer has been halting and slow." Dr. Howard notes further that most new drugs offer only marginal extensions of life and few cures. Additionally, he reports that the new so-called breakthroughs in cancer therapy over promise and under deliver. It's not uncommon for a new, highly advertised cancer drug to cost $10,000 to $30,000 per month, yet may only increase a patient's existence a matter of weeks if it works at all.[19,20]

All too often a promising new cancer drug or procedure is highly touted in reputable scientific journals and reported later that it really doesn't work very well. In fact, in 2015 Dr. Richard Horton, the editor in chief of the *Lancet*, which is considered to be one of the most well respected peer-reviewed medical journals in the world, stated, "The case against science is straightforward: much of the scientific literature, perhaps half, may be simply untrue."[19]

Finally, Dr. Marcia Angell, who recently retired after twenty years as the Editor-in-Chief of the *New England Journal of Medicine* said, "It is simply no longer possible to believe much of the clinical research that is published, or to rely on the judgment of trusted physicians or authoritative medical guidelines. I take no pleasure in this conclusion, which I reached slowly and reluctantly over my two decades as an editor of *The New England Journal of Medicine*."[21,22]

The weather was dreadful several weeks after my last visit with Martha. The temperatures had fallen to well below freezing and northeast Montana experienced blizzards for several days in a row. One afternoon my nurse asked me to step outside of an examination room to talk to someone. She emphasized it was really important. When I stepped out of the examination room,

Georgia directed me to my office where I found a North Dakota Sheriff awaiting me. The man asked me if I had an appointment with Martha that day. I looked at Georgia who told both of us that Martha had an appointment right after lunch, but she did not come. She noted that because of the bad weather and knowing the distance that Martha lived from town, she had just assumed that Martha was delayed and would notify us later. The Sheriff told us that Martha had gone missing and law enforcement and others were trying to find her.

The next day I received a telephone call from Martha's son. He told me a story that in the morning Martha made breakfast for everyone as usual, got all dressed up to come to her doctor's appointment as planned, and after everyone had gone out for their morning activities, they assumed that she drove into town to see me. Near lunchtime a worker noticed that Martha's car was still in the garage and a search started. Unfortunately, late in the day someone found Martha next to her husband's grave by a lake on their property next to a favorite tree. She was dressed in her Sunday best as usual and apparently walked out during the blizzard to be with her husband where she froze to death sitting by the tree. The son just wanted me to know what had happened.

I thanked the son for the telephone call. I thought to myself, "She did it her way, she didn't suffer, and she let Mother Nature take care of her, just like the native Indians. Bless her heart!"

Lars

In the early spring of 1870 during a time of religious perse-
cution and economic hardships in Norway, Bjorn and Ingrid
Larsson, a newlywed pair still in their twenties with a small
child, emigrated from Norway to the United States in search of a
better life. The couple followed many of their countrymen escap-
ing to America in search of freedom, free land, and opportunity.
They traveled from Norway to England where they boarded a
trans-Atlantic ship in Liverpool, England. Then they sailed to
the Port of Québec in Canada. After a few weeks of rest, the newlyweds continued their westward travels overland by ox-drawn
carts, more boats, trains, and wagons. Along the way the pair
met with many fellow Norwegians in Wisconsin and Minnesota
who assisted them with shelter, supplies, and support. In the
early fall they reached their destination and their Norwegian
friends in the Dakota Territory in the United States.

Bjorn and Ingrid found a parcel of land with a good water supply near what would become the Montana and North Dakota bor-
der. Using the provisions of the Homestead Acts they were able to
lay claim to some three hundred twenty acres of free land. Over
the next twenty years the pair had seven more children. As the
children matured Bjorn and Ingrid gave them the original homestead land and claimed additional free land for themselves. The
entire family worked all the homestead farms and prospered. As
the years went by, Bjorn and Ingrid purchased farms of fellow
immigrants who decided to move further west, or who failed farm-
ing, or who died. In time the Larsson family accumulated substantial holdings of property in North Dakota and Montana.

Lars was the eighth and final child born to Bjorn and Ingrid.
He was born quite prematurely in a farmhouse on a wintry day
in the fall of 1898. Lars remembered his mother telling him that
his father weighed him with the milk scale soon after he was

born and he could not have weighed more than two pounds. A shoebox near a wood fired stove served as his crib, and his mother fed him goat's milk with an eyedropper until he was big enough to suck a bottle. Apparently, during the early spring of 1899 a traveling photographer came by their homestead and Ingrid had the man take pictures of the family including Lars in his shoebox on the stove.

All the children grew up on the farm and were educated at a single room schoolhouse several miles from their farm or at home when the weather did not allow them to travel to school. Bjorn and Ingrid made sure that their children obtained as much education as possible in their isolated location. Lars and his siblings all graduated from the eighth grade in the country schoolhouse.

At a community harvest dance when he was a seventeen-year-old boy, Lars met a sixteen-year-old Norwegian girl named Anna Wilhelmsen. Anna and her family owned a farm about twenty miles away from the Larsson family farm. Lars said he could not keep his eyes off this beautiful girl the entire day of the dance. The pair would picnic under a special tree halfway between their two farms during the rest of the fall, and they married before Lars's 18th birthday in the fall of 1916. Using the provisions of the updated Homestead Acts the newlyweds made a claim on three hundred twenty acres of land for their new home.

In the spring of 1917, the United States entered World War I; Lars enlisted in the army and before long he was fighting on the western front in Europe. After two years the war was over, and Lars returned home to Montana and Anna. To his surprise and joy he saw his baby daughter for the first time. Anna had become pregnant just several months before Lars went off to war and Lars was unaware of the child. The Larsson and the Wilhelmsen families worked the farms together during the war so that Lars and Anna could keep their home. Anna would later say that Lars never spoke about the war; he would only say that he was one of the lucky ones who survived long enough to come home.

Armistice Day for World War I was at the 11th hour of the 11th day of the 11th month in 1918. Lars would forevermore celebrate this holiday.

Over the years Lars and Anna had four children. Their first daughter died from diphtheria when she was only four years old as they were traveling through snowdrifts to see a doctor. Later, the pair would have two sons die in World War II and a second daughter would die during childbirth.

Lars and Anna lived and worked on their farm until their early 70s. They then sold it to some neighbors, retired, and moved into the nearest big city, Sidney, Montana.

In late summer of 1977, my nurse Georgia asked if I would be willing to make a home visit to the Larsson's, which was just a few blocks from the clinic. She told me that Mrs. Larsson was ill and that her husband did not want take her to the hospital emergency room. When I asked why they did not just come to the clinic since it was so close, Georgia just informed me that they did not like Sidney doctors. I had heard this comment many times since my arrival in Sidney in 1976, and I promptly asked her to arrange a time for me to visit to their home. Within a short time, Georgia handed me a slip of paper that had the Larsson's address and my anticipated time of arrival, which happened to be after clinic hours that day.

After caring for the last patient in the clinic I traveled the short distance to the Larsson home. An elderly man greeted me at the front door, promptly extended his hand, and said his name was Lars Larsson. He thanked me for coming and told me briefly that his wife of over sixty years had a fever and a severe backache. He told me that he had been unable to get her to take sips of liquids, and she had not had a meal in several days. He took me into their bedroom where an elderly lady was resting. Lars introduced me to his wife Anna.

After a short examination I concluded that Anna was most likely suffering from a urinary track infection that had progressed up into her kidneys. Dehydration from not drinking fluids was complicating the situation. I advised the pair of my thoughts and offered to put Anna in the hospital for treatment. The couple respectfully declined my offer. They told me that patients only went to the hospital in Sidney to die, and they would have no part of that.

I certainly had a dilemma on my hands. At the time there was no such thing as home nursing care. Some considered treating people at home without professional nursing care unethical, and it certainly was not condoned in our small community by the medical establishment.

Historically, families have cared for their disabled and sick loved ones at home with perhaps some distant direction from someone in the medical field. Beginning sometime in the mid 1800s, nurses making periodic visits to homes filled a niche that was needed to care for the sick and injured as well as provide information on such topics as newborn care and prenatal care. However, most of the home nursing care visits were done on a volunteer basis and were not readily available in all locations.

A significant change occurred in 1911 when the Metropolitan Life Insurance Company became the first company to pay for visiting nurse services for their policyholders. Soon thereafter other companies followed with similar programs; home care nursing services companies started up everywhere.

When hospital-based care became dominant beginning in the 1930s, the development of home care services diminished. This produced three tiers of service for sick patients: hospital-based care, home-based community services care, and private pay care.

The landscape changed in 1965 with the Medicare legislation that provided payment for home care benefits for the elderly. Over the next fifty years with a reliable payment source, home healthcare services expanded significantly. Compensation for home care now includes payments not only for nurses but also for physical and occupational therapists, nutritionists, social workers, respiratory therapists, and many more.

In addition to Medicare and Medicaid payments, many insurance companies now allow their clients to receive part or all of their life insurance or long-term-care benefits early to pay for home care services.[23,24]

I knew, however, that Anna would recover with some fluids and some antibiotics. Therefore, I asked the pair if they would be willing to allow me to treat Anna at home, and I described what I would be doing with the treatment. After a short pause they agreed.

I returned to my clinic where I gathered up the medications and materials that I thought would be needed to treat Anna. Georgia was still at the clinic assisting the other doctors. I informed her of my predicament and asked if she would be willing to help me. Enthusiastically she agreed. Georgia had recently graduated from nursing school and was excited about anything involving nursing. Together we returned to the Larsson home to begin Anna's treatment.

My first task was to obtain blood samples for evaluation. Next Georgia inserted a catheter into Anna's bladder to obtain a sterile urine specimen for evaluation and a culture. Since Georgia was a new nurse and needed the experience, I allowed her to insert an intravenous catheter in Anna's arm and connect it to a bag of fluid. Through the intravenous line we started a broad-spectrum antibiotic that I anticipated changing once the urine cultures were completed. Lars was given the jobs of making sure the intravenous line continued to function and that the bag of fluid did not run empty. Additionally, Lars was instructed to take and record Anna's temperature every few hours. He was given instructions to have the hospital contact me if he had any issues. Georgia and I then left to take the samples to the hospital laboratory.

The following morning I went to the Larsson home before going to the hospital to see how Anna was doing. I noticed that a second bottle of intravenous fluid had been started and Lars informed me that Georgia had come about midnight to check on

Anna and exchanged IV fluid bottles. Anna looked a lot better and her fever had abated. She was sitting up in bed, and Lars was feeding her some chicken soup. Everybody knows that chicken soup is good for every illness.

Georgia checked Anna over her lunch break that day and added another intravenous fluid bottle. By mid afternoon the laboratory urine culture reports returned and showed that Anna's antibiotic treatment was appropriate. After clinic hours Georgia and I made another visit to the Larsson home together. Anna was dramatically better than she was the day before. We told Lars and Anna that we would continue with the treatment for another day and then Anna could take antibiotic pills. They both expressed their appreciation to us for our efforts.

Georgia checked in on Anna again during the evening and added yet another bottle of intravenous fluid. The following morning when I visited I laid out a plan of care for the next ten days that included antibiotic pills and repeat urine tests in a few days. That evening I brought the antibiotic pills to Anna and removed her IV.

Before I could leave that evening, Lars set me down to have a chat. It was at this time that he revealed to me the history of his family coming to America. Lars then pulled out of his wallet a tattered black-and-white photo encased in a yellowish plastic sleeve revealing a small baby in a shoebox asleep on a wood fired stove. He told me that was his picture. As I was leaving Lars asked me to accompany him into his massive vegetable garden. With a paper bag in his hand he collected fresh tomatoes, corn, squash, and beans for me to take home. This was the first time I received payment other than money for my services. A short time later Lars telephoned my office and left a message that Anna was back to her old self.

On a spring morning about three years later Georgia received another message from Lars who asked that we come to see Anna at their home. The message was that Anna wasn't able to speak. Again, Lars did not want to take his wife to the hospital because he repeated, "That's where people die in Sidney, Montana." After Lars assured Georgia that Anna was in no acute distress and in no immediate danger, she told him that she and the doctor would come over at lunchtime in a few hours. We visited the Larsson home over lunch and found Anna lying in bed. Not only could she not speak but also she had no movement on the left side of her body. I told Lars that Anna obviously had a stroke sometime during the night that paralyzed the left side of her body. I encouraged him to let us have the ambulance transport her to the hospital. He declined. He informed us that they had taken care of each other for almost sixty-five years, and he was not going to stop now. He just wanted to know what he could do.

I told him frankly that his wife had a good chance of dying within the first few weeks after a major stroke. If she did survive, the chances were very good that one side of her body would not work and her mental function would be abnormal. He thanked me for my candor; he just wanted to know the truth and what he could expect.

Thereafter, either Georgia or I visited the Larsson home twice a day because there was no visiting nurse service available in Sidney, Montana, at the time. Anna never really improved and remained unconscious. Lars remained at Anna's side day and night for the next two weeks until she died.

Afterward Lars was never the same. He did not plant his big garden that year and let the ground grow up in weeds. Through the summer I would occasionally go by his home to see how he was doing; Lars would never complain. I could see, however, that he was quite sad and lonely. In mid fall of that year Lars developed an upper respiratory illness I believed was most likely influenza. As the illness progressed I offered to place Lars in the hospital. He declined. He just wanted to stay at home. Again, Georgia and I started visiting Lars twice a day at his home. His illness intensified which caused him to have even worse respiratory difficulty. Subsequently, either Georgia or I visited him every four hours because Lars always refused to go to the hospital. One

morning Georgia came into my clinic office and told me that Lars
had told her that he was ready to meet Anna. He asked Georgia
to shave his face; she did. He also had Georgia open his bedroom
window, which I learned was a Scandinavian tradition to allow
the soul to escape to its loved ones. Lars was near death, and
Georgia thought that I should visit him over lunch. The hospice
movement had not yet come to our community in 1980.

Historically, hospice referred to a place of rest and hospital-
ity for travelers in Europe. A physician in England named Dame
Cicely Saunders worked extensively with the terminally ill in
London, started the St. Christopher's Hospice in London in
1967, and is generally credited with founding the modern hospice movement. Many things happened over the next two
decades in American government regarding medical care resulting in the 1986 legislation that made end-of-life hospice benefits
permanent for Medicare and Medicaid recipients. Soon thereafter programs for palliative care, which were originally
intended to relieve the suffering of terminally ill patients,
became focused on other chronic disabling conditions such as
respiratory disease, chronic pain, and psychiatric disorders such
as severe anxiety.[25,26]

Before I went to Lars' home that noontime, I called the local
mortuary to inform the mortician, who was also the county corner, about Lars's situation and that he might die at home that
day. The mortician told me not to worry because Lars has made
all the arrangements in advance as if he knew his days were
numbered.

When I visited Lars at noon he asked me to sit at his bedside.
After I pulled up a chair beside him, he took out the old tattered
picture of that little baby in a shoebox on a wood stove. He said,
"That little guy did okay didn't he Doc?"

I nodded my head in agreement.

By now Lars was struggling with every breath. He picked up
a picture of Anna as a young woman and said he would be with
her soon. Grabbing for my hand and whispering between gasping

breaths Lars asked me not to leave him because he didn't want to die alone. I assured him I would be with him.

Lars died quietly in his sleep about half an hour later. I called the mortician so he could fulfill the remainder of Lars' wishes. I then called Georgia to let her know that Lars had died and asked her to reschedule my appointments for the afternoon because I was taking the rest of the day off. Georgia was already way ahead of me as usual by knowing I needed a mental break. She told me that all the patients were rescheduled and that I should go home to drive my tractor for a while.

As I was leaving the clinic, I suggested to Georgia that she also take the rest of the day off to be with her little kids.

I Can't Walk

In the mid 1850s a French physician named Landry described a condition in which the patient had an acute onset of peripheral muscle paralysis that rapidly progressed from the feet to near total muscle paralysis below the mid chest area over a period of several hours. The paralysis was not associated with any infectious disease and the symptoms resolved over a period of six months or so without any noticeable residual muscular weakness. This disorder presented very much like polio except that polio was known to be associated with an infectious disease and there was always some type of muscle wasting and functional loss if the patient survived the initial infection. This new disorder was named *Landry's paralysis* or *French polio*.

In 1916, two French doctors, George Guillain and Jean Alexandria Barré, diagnosed a similar illness in several soldiers. These French physicians were able to discern and describe the key diagnostic abnormality in this illness, an interesting combination of findings in the spinal fluid of a normal cell count and an increase in spinal fluid protein. Since they had no idea about the cause of the illness, the doctors had no treatment. They could only observe the patient and record their findings.

One hundred twenty years later the United States was engaged in the Vietnam War. During the 1970s, many of our military personnel returned to United States with a variety of curious illnesses that were rarely seen in this country. In 1973, the neurology department at the Veterans Administration Hospital in Portland, Oregon, received young infantrymen from Vietnam with a similar syndrome of rapidly increasing muscle paralysis over a few hours to a few days time for no apparent reason. During a single three-week interval, seven cases were admitted to the Veterans Hospital in Portland. I happened to be on the neurology service as a senior medical student during this time. The neurology resident counseled me to observe these patients carefully because I probably would never see similar cases again. The doctor said all the patients had a rare disorder called Guillain-Barré syndrome. Additionally, he said that the usual incidence of this disorder in the regular population was approximately one case in a million people per year. Normally, the Portland Veterans Administration Hospital would see a similar patient every year or two. Now the resident doctor had seven cases of Guillain-Barré syndrome in three weeks all coming from Viet Nam.

Just like Dr. Landry a century before, the neurology resident taught me that we still had no idea what caused the disease or how to treat it. Our treatment of these young men was careful observation. We did know, however, that approximately twenty-five to fifty percent of the patients would have a paralysis that would progress up into the chest muscles resulting in respiratory failure. Only then were we able to provide any significant treatment by placing the patient on a ventilator in the intensive care unit. Over the next weeks to months one of the patients died from respiratory failure, but the others fortunately survived their illnesses. Unfortunately after six months over half of the survivors had various residual neurologic dysfunctions including difficulty walking, chronic pain, fatigue, and muscle weakness.

Landry-Guillain-Barré syndrome is a collection of neurologic findings that occurs in all seasons and affects both children and adults of all ages. Males are affected about 1.5 times more often than females and adults are affected slightly more than children. Its cause is unknown but it produces an acute, severe inflammation response in the body that targets certain and variable nerve groups; all attempts to date to isolate a specific virus or other microbial agent have been unsuccessful. Perhaps there are multiple causes for Guillain-Barré and our perpetual searching for simple solutions to complex problems has confused medical researchers. Although many cases are concurrent with or preceded by a viral infection, no single organism has been isolated.

Despite tremendous progress over the years in our laboratory sciences, the mainstay for diagnosis remains the abnormalities in spinal fluid first appreciated by Drs. Guillain and Barré in the early 1900s. At the turn of the twenty-first century no reliable treatment had been discovered for this disorder.[27,28,29,30]

Almost fifteen years after my medical school experience in neurology, I examined a teenage boy brought into the Sidney hospital emergency department from a nearby rural community. The boy complained of pain in his legs and an inability to walk that had started just the night before. He said his legs felt like dough. The teenager had not been sick or injured in anyway that he or the family members could recall. For all the parents knew he was a vigorous young farm boy in his normal good state of health who got sick all of a sudden. By the time I saw the boy for the first time, he had leg muscle paralysis below his knees. He complained of his feet being asleep but not totally without feeling. The reflexes at his knees and ankles were absent. Examinations of his heart, lungs, and abdomen were unremarkable. His mental status was good. His blood tests were absolutely normal. I knew I had seen this pattern before in medical school, and I was convinced that my young patient had Guillain-Barré syndrome. After consultation with the local internal medicine physician and a regional neurologist, we jointly confirmed the diagnosis and decided to admit the teenager to our hospital for observation. Over the next few days the muscle paralysis progressed upward to the mid chest area, but respiratory problems were never encountered. Our patient was unable to walk or even roll over in bed because the muscles in his legs did not work. I performed a spinal tap, a procedure using a long needle that is inserted between the vertebra in the back penetrating near the spinal cord to retrieve a sample of spinal fluid. Upon analysis the fluid revealed the classic findings of *French polio* of increased protein and normal blood cells, the same findings made by the French doctors Guillain and Dr. Barré in the early 1900s. Just like Doctor Landry in the mid 19th-century or any other physician up to that point in time, the consultants and I had no idea what caused the disorder or how to treat it. However, I did know that a certain number these patients would die from respiratory failure so I made sure that this department was on alert at all times and its therapists performed pulmonary function tests multiple times each day. At no time during the patient's hospitalization did my young patient develop a need for their services, thank goodness.

The teenager remained in the hospital for several weeks. Despite the pain and fear of being unable to walk, he never complained. The physical therapists frequently noted that our patient was a real trooper while he was undergoing painful therapy sessions. The paralysis gradually descended to the point he could walk with crutches, and the sensation in his legs improved dramatically. We discharged the young man from the hospital to his home with a program for extensive physical therapy knowing that he may or may not have residual muscular weakness and may not walk normally again.

About a year and a half later I watched this young man participate in football, basketball, and track events as a high school senior. I noticed he still had a small limp, but this did not deter him from giving his full effort. I could not help but smile and applaud his every athletic effort.

Few people would ever know how sick this boy had been or how far he had come from his days of near total muscular paralysis, but I did. I hoped he would have a bright future.

A Hometown Hero

Mr. Walter Raymond came into my office one morning in the fall. He was one of the patriarchs of the community and was my son's adviser in a youth program. I had never seen Mr. Raymond as patient even though I had been in the community over twenty years. Therefore, I was a bit surprised to see him since he normally saw one of the internal medicine doctors in town.

Mr. Raymond explained to me that he had a tickle in his throat and a raspy voice for several months. The first doctor he saw told him that he had a mild viral infection of his vocal cords and prescribed a course of antibiotics. (Antibiotics do nothing for viral infections.) When his symptoms did not resolve after a month or so, he went to see another physician because his primary physician was on vacation. This doctor told him he had laryngitis and that he should have voice rest for least two weeks. He was given a regimen of gargles with salt water several times a day. Again, his symptoms did not resolve. Finally Walter came to see me for a third opinion because he felt something was not right, and he wanted to get to the bottom of it.

After taking a more comprehensive history, which was unremarkable except that he was a perpetual pipe smoker, I palpated Mr. Raymond's neck. I found multiple hard, non-tender lymph nodes that were fixed to the underlying tissues and certainly had been there for some time. A cursory examination of his throat and palpation in his mouth with my fingers did not reveal any obvious abnormality. Performing indirect laryngoscopy, a maneuver that requires using a light source and a hand held mirror on a stick to view the vocal cords with reflected light, I was overcome with a sickening feeling when I saw an obvious growth above, below, and around the vocal cords that looked very much like a cauliflower. I observed that one side of the vocal cords was not moving which was most likely caused by damage to the nerves by the tumor. With the enlarged lymph nodes in his neck, my strong suspicion was that he had an advanced cancer of his throat. I told Mr. Raymond that I saw something I didn't like and suggested that he should see Doctor Arbor, our community's ear nose and throat specialist. When he acquiesced to my suggestion, I telephoned the physician's office that was just down the hallway. I spoke with Dr. Arbor, told him what I thought I saw, and asked if he could see Mr. Raymond soon.

Dr. Arbor told me to send the patient immediately to his office.

Late that afternoon Dr. Arbor called to tell me that my suspicions were correct. With his better equipment, he could see that the tumor was more extensive than my cursory evaluation revealed. He congratulated me on finding the tumor saying that in his experience most primary care physicians did not know how to use a laryngeal mirror to evaluate the throat below the tongue onto the vocal cords. The doctor also told me he had taken the liberty of taking pictures of the lesion, showing them to Mr. Raymond and arranging for him to see a radiation therapist in the next day or so. Dr. Arbor did not think the lesion was something that could be operated upon because of its size and its spread. Our patient had stage IV throat cancer.[31,32]

About a week later Mr. Raymond returned to my clinic just to talk. He needed some advice regarding further treatment for the lesion in his throat. He related what Dr. Arbor had told him and what the radiation cancer doctor had told him regarding treatment. However, the doctors were pretty vague on its effectiveness or the adverse effects. He was told that his life expectancy was twelve months or less without treatment. If he had a good result from radiation this might be extended for perhaps another year.

Mr. Raymond asked me quietly if I knew he had throat cancer when I first examined him. I told him that I thought he did, but I was not an expert in the field and that a biopsy was needed to confirm the diagnosis. I did not want to tell him something awful that turned out to be not true. He thanked me for my honesty.

Mr. Raymond said that his wife whom he had been caring for at home for several years had increasing dementia, and he knew she could not take care of herself. He also told me that his children had been estranged from him and his wife for some time so he did not think they were willing to take care of their mother if he was gone. Essentially, he wanted to know how long he had to get things in order before he died. He was asking me to make his end-of-life decisions because he was convinced his family could not. He just wanted to know what to do.

I suggested to Mr. Raymond that he get his affairs in order before he started any treatment because the radiation was going to make him very weak, and he may have difficulty concentrating. Additionally, he should expect a lot of pain and the chances were good that he would not survive any longer with treatment. Mr. Raymond told me he didn't think he would have any more treatment for the cancer. Again, he thanked me for my candor and left the clinic.

Somebody has to make decisions about a patient's death and dying wishes. As a physician, I had to assume this responsibility more times than I wish to remember because the affected parties could not or refused to make decisions regarding end-of-life care. In the late 1970s financial planners and lawyers started a concerted effort to get people to make end-of-life decisions while they were mentally intact. Hospitals attempted to have patients file their personal powers of attorney and living will documents with them to avoid their receiving unnecessary and unwanted heroic measures should something adverse occur during a hospitalization. All of these efforts proved minimally successful for a variety of reasons. The biggest reason was that the client, or the patient, did not want to discuss death and dying issues while they were alive. Indeed, few people entering hospitals have their end-of-life wishes documented in their medical records. In the past the price to produce end-of-life documents was a concern because the

process required professional assistance from a lawyer or a financial planner. Now, however, with the development of the microcomputer and the internet, people can access these forms
through online legal sources for minimal expense. Still only a
small percentage of people take advantage of the services.

Additionally, end-of-life decisions made in advance are frequently modified by the wishes of family members, a change in
family circumstances, or the dying patient. All too often I have
seen dying patient's family members make decisions about what
they wanted that were contrary to what their loved one wanted.
All too often I witnessed dying patients submit to chemotherapy
or radical surgeries in vain attempts to pacify family members.

Having personally attended many dying patients, I know
that a significant number of end-of-life decisions are made at the
bedside as a loved one is about to succumb. Perhaps this is the
way the end of life was meant to be, but often it makes for a legal
quagmire for the family after the loved one is gone.

For the next few months as news of Mr. Raymond's illness
spread to the community, accolades for his accomplishments
poured in. He received the lifetime achievement award from the
International Kiwanis organization. Multiple events were held in
his honor. He took in all this adulation with the same low-key
approach he had to life and gave all the credit for any of his
accomplishments to others. He told me he was touched by all the
fuss but a bit embarrassed.

Because of his work with a local youth program and the
development of young boys over a period of twenty to thirty
years, there was an initiative to develop a scholarship program in
his name for the boys graduating from high school. This idea had
started in the fall before anyone knew about Mr. Raymond's illness, but his medical issues precluded his being an active partic-
ipant in the development process. Perhaps six months after
seeing Mr. Raymond in my office I went to his home to ask his
permission for the scholarship program in his name. Walter was
sitting in his chair covered with a blanket because he was cold

even though the house was very warm. He was ashen in color and appeared near death.

Barely able to speak, Walter whispered to me that initially he wasn't going to have any treatment for his cancer, but to keep peace within the family he agreed to radiation therapy. He told me he had not felt well since the first treatment and knew then he was not going to last much longer. Mr. Raymond was not afraid to die, but he was most concerned about his wife's future because of her dementia. When I talked to him about the proposed scholarship program, Walter smiled, chuckled to himself, and started to cry. He told me he couldn't think of a better way to spend other peoples' money than to help young people. He agreed to present the first scholarships in a few weeks at the annual graduation for the youth program.

As I left his home that day I thought that Mr. Raymond's immune system must have been near the breaking point when I first saw him. After a course of radiation therapy that put further stresses on his system, his body could not handle the additional insult. His immune system succumbed, and the cancer spread rapidly.

Over the next few weeks Mr. Raymond deteriorated quickly. Despite the amount of pain I knew that he had, he did not complain. That was his way.

He died about nine months after the original diagnosis was made and just several days before the scholarship ceremony where the first awards were given in his honor. Mourners from across United States came to his funeral in our small town to pay their last respects to this humble hero.

The Catheter

We had been in Sidney, Montana, just a short time when one day my family and I went shopping at the local department store. Since this was a small store, it was common for the product you wished to purchase not to be in stock and the customer had to submit a mail order. Such it was on this occasion, and I was at the mail order counter. After the attendant completed my request she asked if I was the new doctor in town. When I told her that I was indeed new in town and that my office was in the Medical Arts Clinic, she asked if I made house calls. When I replied that I would make a home visit if she would give me some specifics. The woman introduced herself as Margaret and told me that she had a very sick husband. She worked only a few hours a day because she had to care for him at home. Her husband did not have insurance nor could he get insurance because of his illness. They had already consumed all of their savings and had re-mortgaged their home to pay for his medical bills. Her husband's usual doctor was the elder physician in town who was away for a few weeks, and none of the other local doctors were willing to see her husband unless she took him to their clinic and paid for the visit at that time. Margaret stated that moving her husband caused him a lot of pain, she could not move him by herself, and she could not pay for an ambulance to take him to the hospital just a few blocks away. The woman told me her husband had just called her at work to tell her that he was having severe pain again. Margaret wanted to know if I would be willing to see her husband at their home.

I agreed.

She gave me her address and I consented to come as soon as I took my family back to our home in the country. In the early afternoon I pulled up to the modest ranch style house on the west edge of town. I did not know what to expect since I had not yet obtained a more formal history of the gentleman's problem.

Margaret answered the door and welcomed me inside. I cannot explain it, but the smell of death was inside the building. There was an odor that I had experienced before only in areas where someone was dying. I could hear moaning coming from a room further inside the home. Suddenly a man's voice was crying complaining of severe pain. Margaret escorted me into the bedroom where her husband was resting. He was a man of not yet sixty years but with his sunken eyes and sallow face he appeared much older and near death. At this point Margaret told me that her husband had cancer and had only short time to live. However, for the time that he did have left, she wanted him to be as comfortable as possible. The pain pills she had been giving him did not seem to be working. She implored me to help if I could.

I introduced myself to Arthur, the husband, who despite his severe pain and agony, was able to give me a smile and welcomed me to his home. Arthur was unable to provide any more history but agreed to let me examine him.

His skin was yellowish. The conjunctivas of his eyes were yellow. This is called jaundice, and it told me that his liver was either not working or was obstructed. His lungs were just full of noises that definitely were not normal. His heart examination, however, was unremarkable. An examination of his abdomen revealed multiple masses. In his upper right abdomen there was a hard lumpy mass where his liver should be that was obviously cancerous. It was not tender to touch, and I assumed it was most likely the reason for his jaundice. The second mass all along his left abdomen felt like a hard lumpy rope about three inches wide stretching from Arthur's ribs to his pelvis. This was his large intestine full of hard stool. Margaret told me she thought her husband had had a bowel movement perhaps a week before. Constipation is a common finding when patients take a lot of narcotic pain medicine. This mass also was not tender to touch. Finally, there was a mass the size of a small volleyball just above his pelvic bone that was extremely tender to touch and was definitely the cause of the man's immediate pain. I knew this was his severely distended bladder and it needed to be drained soon. Margaret told me she had no idea when Arthur urinated last.

I commented that her husband's bladder had to be drained with a catheter. I offered to put him in the hospital to do this, but Margaret declined and begged me to help her husband at home. I agreed, but first I had to go to the hospital a few blocks away to get the necessary supplies.

At the hospital I talked with Elizabeth Clawson, RN who was the charge nurse of the day. This nurse had been around the block a few times in medicine and would prove in the coming years to be a wonderful resource for my continuing education in rural medicine. Elizabeth gathered up the appropriate supplies I requested for the procedure. As I was about to pick up the materials and leave she said, "Doctor, just wait a minute." Elizabeth told me she was going to get something else that I might need, just in case. When I asked what that might be she replied, "The filiform catheters."

When I was in medical school many of my classmates thought that performing menial tasks while taking care of patients was below them. For goodness sakes, they were going to be doctors, not orderlies or nurses. They referred to tasks such as inserting intravenous lines, drawing blood samples, inserting bladder catheters, changing bandages, and others as scut work. I, however, always enjoyed doing this work because it always included procedures that needed to be done to take care of our patients, the work was necessary, and it gave me good experience that I might use later. Additionally, I learned that the more I was willing to perform menial tasks to take care of our patients, the more responsibility the attending interns, residents, and faculty would allow me when more difficult procedures needed to be performed.

When I was doing my urology rotation at the Portland Veterans Administration Hospital, my senior resident was Doctor Skip Edwards. One day we were called to the emergency department at the hospital for a patient with acute urinary retention. The emergency room doctor reported that the nurses had attempted to insert a catheter but had been unsuccessful. Therefore, it became the duty for the urology department to manage the patient. Some of my colleagues called this a dump. I called it another learning opportunity. Dr. Edwards and I made our way to the emergency room to see the patient, a seventy-year-old World War II veteran who was having a tremendous amount of pain in his abdomen. Dr. Edwards asked the man if he had had any previous episodes of difficulty urinating. The man told us that he had bladder cancer that was being treated by doctors at the Wadsworth Veterans Hospital in California and he was just on vacation visiting family in Oregon. When asked, he told us that he urinated just fine the day before.

Dr. Edwards surmised that the tumor had gotten big enough to obstruct the section of the man's urethra within the prostate gland and suggested that we attempt to put in another bladder catheter. He asked the nurse to retrieve a certain size urinary catheter and put it in the freezer compartment of the refrigerator for a few minutes. Dr. Edwards explained that this was a little trick to make the catheter firmer and stiffer. After a few minutes the nurse brought the frozen urinary bladder catheter, which Doctor Edwards attempted to insert. The attempt was unsuccessful because the man's urinary channel was too small. Dr. Edwards asked me to attempt to put in the catheter because, as he always said, "It's a teaching hospital." As expected, my attempt failed too. Dr. Edwards requested that the nurse bring him a set of filiform catheters. When I asked what filiform catheters were, he just asked me to be patient and wait-and-see. After a short wait, during which we were reassuring the patient that we would relieve his pain soon, the nurse returned with a small, sterilized package from surgery with a label on top: FILI-FORM CATHETER SET. Dr. Edwards opened the package and showed me that the first catheter piece, called the introducer, had no hole in it. It was quite stiff, about eight inches long, and the size of a pencil lead in diameter with a well-rounded tip. The other end had metal threads for attaching sequentially larger catheters with holes in them. The idea behind the instrument was that once the urinary channel had been dilated to an appropriate size, a regular balloon bladder catheter could be inserted. Once Dr. Edwards had explained the instrument to me he said, "Jim, have at it." He then gave me step-by-step instructions on how to safely insert the filiform catheters. When I completed the procedure, we allowed the man's bladder to drain clear yellow urine, which promptly relieved his pain. Then I removed the filiform catheter and reinserted a large, frozen ballooned bladder catheter, which is also called a Foley catheter. Afterward, an orderly transported our patient to the urology ward for observation.

When nurse Elizabeth returned with the filiform catheter kit I put it into the bag with the rest of my materials and headed back to Margaret's home to care for Arthur. My initial attempt to insert a regular urinary catheter into Arthur's bladder was unsuccessful because of an obstruction between Arthur's penis and his bladder. Now Margaret told me that she remembered her husband had urinated the previous evening. This confirmed that there was indeed a tract still open into the man's bladder. Therefore, I opened up the filiform catheter set and slowly but gently inserted the very small lead guide for the catheter. Fortunately, I was able to push the lead tip into the bladder without difficulty as evidenced by urine leaking around it. Then in sequence I added increasingly larger catheter sizes onto the lead catheter until I had a generous flow of urine from Arthur's bladder. I allowed the urine to drain slowly into a bag over a period of a few minutes. As soon as the pressure in Arthur's bladder was diminished, he stopped moaning. Eventually about two thousand milliliters, or about two quarts, of urine came out of his bladder.

After the bladder drained I performed a rectal exam and found what I expected, hard impacted stool. With a gloved hand, I started to gently extract the hard pieces of stool from the man's rectum. After I had pulled out perhaps two handfuls of stool,

Arthur had a massive bowel movement onto the bed. The mass on the left side of his abdomen was now on the bed and the room smelled awful. Fortunately, I had placed paper drapes under the man before I started this procedure and Margaret and I were able to clean up in short order. Margaret must have used an entire can of bathroom deodorizer to remove the stench. I suggested that she take another can of deodorizer and walk through her home to deodorize the entire home. Afterward, Arthur was comfortable and no longer moaning. Two of the three masses in his abdomen we're gone. I knew it was the tumor in his liver that would eventually kill him, but not today. Our job was to make Arthur more comfortable, and Margaret and I succeeded.

I jotted down a note outlining what we had done for Margaret to give to her husband's usual physician when he returned from his vacation. I instructed Margaret to give her husband a water enema every two days to make sure he did not get obstructed with stool again. Before I left, I exchanged the filiform catheter with a regular balloon type catheter that could stay in an extended time. Unlike today's disposable medical supply system, the filiform catheter set was not disposable and had to be returned to the hospital's surgery department for sterilization and reuse.

Arthur's family doctor never called or communicated to me in any way. Much to my dismay, I learned that this lack of communication between physicians not only within our community but also with the outlying communities was the norm in the region during my beginning years of medical practice in Sidney, Montana.

Beginning in the late 1980s medical care facilities of all types started to computerize. Without any uniformity in computer systems and programs, communication between competing doctors and competing hospitals within the same community and across state boundaries was at best a perplexing situation and at worst a quagmire of confusion. Over the next two decades Congress passed national legislation first encouraging, and then mandating, electronic medical records. Acronyms for the laws such as HIPPA (Health Information Privacy and Portability Act), the ACA (the Affordable Care Act or Obamacare), and others pressed the concept of an electronic medical record for each citizen that was easily transferable no matter where the person was. With mandates from the Affordable Care Act that all citizens with few exceptions were required to have health insurance, Congress had the idea that minimal cost health insurance for all citizens added to a universal, easily accessible personalized electronic record would make people healthier. How they came up with these ideas is anyone's guess. Insurance and computers do not and cannot make people healthier.

To date the only thing that can be shown for certain is that the electronic medical record improves billing and accounting services. There is no evidence that computerization of patient records has made a significant improvement in patient morbidity rates (the number of people hurt or injured) and patient mortality rates (the number of deaths). Theoretically every patient should now have access to all of his or her medical records via a computer terminal. For legal reasons I am confident few people, if any, have access to a complete set of their medical records.[33]

Some months later I met Margaret again at the local department store. She told me that Arthur had died at home peacefully just a few weeks after my visit. She thanked me again for taking care of him during his time of need. Margaret asked when she could expect a bill for my services. I knew that she was already having difficulty paying her bills so I told her that watching her husband become comfortable again was enough payment for me.

She motioned with her arm for me to come around the counter so she could give me a hug. She gave me a big hug with a big thank-you. Some payments we doctors receive are far more valuable than money.

The Biker

Ezra Montgomery was just making ends meet in San Francisco in the spring of 1979 when he heard about the North Dakota oil boom and the plentiful jobs in the Williston basin in eastern Montana and western North Dakota. Since he had recently been divorced and had no particular family ties to anyone in California, Ezra decided late one night during a bout of drinking with his buddies that he was going to the oilfields to make his fortune. The next morning he loaded a few of his clothes, hopped on his Harley-Davidson motorcycle, and headed to Montana.

Ezra had never been very reliable for working a real job. In fact, his lack of constant employment was the primary reason for his divorce. His wife called him a lazy bum. Sometime during his trip to Montana Ezra decided that he should be a truck driver since he heard they made really good money and they could sleep in their trucks. When Ezra got to the Bakken oil fields he promptly started to look for truck driving jobs, but to his surprise he soon learned that before he could drive a truck he needed to have a Department of Transportation or DOT certificate. This required a physical examination so he could get the card that allowed him to learn how to drive a truck followed by taking the truck drivers' examinations. When he passed all of these hurdles, then, and only then, could he try to find someone willing to employ him. Ezra came to my clinic for his DOT examination.

An interesting part of his history was that Ezra had rheumatic fever as a child, developed diseased heart valves, and had a mitral valve replaced in his heart about six years before. During the examination I asked Ezra how he came to Sidney, Montana. After he told me his story, I asked if he knew how to drive a truck. Ezra replied, "Hey Doc, if I can ride a Harley, I can surely drive a truck." Despite being about fifty pounds overweight and having click-clap noticeable noises on his heart exam made by his mechanical heart valve, Ezra met the physical requiremerts for the DOT license, which I issued.

The first frost in northeastern Montana frequently comes in the early part of September. From that time until the spring thaw in March or April inclement weather can happen anytime. Early one Saturday evening in early fall just after suppertime I was summoned to the emergency room. It was really cold this evening with the temperature near 0°. Kathy, the charge nurse on duty, told me there had been a motorcycle accident about thirty miles south of town where the highway winds through a hilly area near a town called Intake.

The volunteer ambulance crew reported that their patient, who had been riding a big Harley-Davidson motorcycle that went off the icy road, was having chills they attributed to hypothermia. They noticed that the patient was confused and could not give any history about the accident suggesting a head injury. The ambulance reported that the man had been placed on a spine board and his neck had been stabilized with a cervical collar per EMS (Emergency Medical Systems) protocol. Apparently, by gross evaluation of the accident scene, the man's motorcycle veered off the road and hit an embankment. The rider, who was not wearing a protective helmet, catapulted about sixty feet onto the side of a hill. The ambulance was transporting their patient with utmost speed, which meant to me that the driver, as usual, was exceeding the speed limit appropriate for the road conditions.

I reached the emergency room a few minutes before the ambulance when Kathy told me there were no updates on the patient's condition. In addition, she said the warming blankets were ready if the patient was hypothermic.

When the victim was brought into the emergency room his cold, damp clothing was removed promptly with scissors. Our patient was a massive man who was indeed shivering, but his vital signs revealed that his temperature was 101°. His pulse was rapid and his blood pressure was low normal. These were not the physical signs of someone who was hypothermic but rather the findings of someone who was infected and septic. I had to change my thinking pattern quickly from caring for a hypothermic trauma patient to a severely infected patient with unknown trauma.

The man was barely responsive to voice commands. When I asked his name, he gave a woman's name. When asked if he knew where he was, the man replied, "Canada." When asked if he knew what date it was, he said it was the 4th of July. Finally, when I asked him if he knew who the president of the United States was, he replied, "George Washington." Obviously, the man was confused which could have been from head trauma, infection, drugs, or a whole host of reasons. Therefore, I knew the man needed to be examined thoroughly from head to toe.

Except for a few abrasions on his head, I found no obvious abnormalities from his accident. However, his right pupil was dilated and reacted slowly to light stimulation which is sometimes seen after direct trauma to the eye. The left pupil was smaller and reacted poorly. The left upper eyelid had a slight droop. The confused man could not cooperate with me so I could not test his eye motion. I found no obvious bleeding or abnormalities in the man's ears, nose, or throat.

The external chest had been protected by clothing and had no abrasions or deformities. There was a mid-sternal scar that was well healed indicating that the man had had chest surgery in the past. Everyone in that emergency room could easily hear without a stethoscope the swoosh-click-swoosh-click sounds from the man's artificial heart valve. The heart valve noise was significant but with my stethoscope it was easy for me to hear a significant heart murmur. The patient's lungs were grossly clear when he took a deep breath. His abdomen was massive, but I found no obvious masses, scars, or areas of tenderness. The man's arms had a few abrasions from the accident that I deemed insignificant, but needle tracks were easily visible with multiple pustules indicating infection from recent injections, most likely containing illegal drugs. On his palms and fingers I found small red bumps called Janeway lesions and small petechial hemorrhages called splinter hemorrhages which are usually diagnostic of an infection in the heart called bacterial endocarditis, a really bad condition for someone with an artificial heart valve. My thought process quickly changed again to sepsis caused by illegal drug use in a man with an artificial heart valve.[34,35,36]

Before I continued my examination I asked the charge nurse to have the laboratory technician obtain some blood not only for the usual trauma panel of tests but also for cultures of the man's blood.

My continued examination revealed no gross deformities or abnormalities of the man's legs or genitalia. A rectal exam revealed no gross blood or perforations.

A brief neurological evaluation of the legs revealed grossly normal reflexes at the knees and the ankles. Stimulation of the left foot on the outer edge with a blunt object, known as a Babinski reflex test, produced a downward deviation of the toes, a normal response. The same test on the right foot, however, produced an abnormal response with the great toe pointing upward. I remembered the words of one of my British neurology mentors in medical school after he encountered a similar response on one of our hospital patients, "Alas, my young doctor, there is something terribly amiss in this patient's noggin."

This event occurred in the days before CT scans, MRI scans, and 3-D cardiac echocardiography. Diagnosis and treatment decisions had to be made on what the doctor could see and touch and what the doctor thought was happening inside his patient's body. I knew within the first few minutes of this man's arrival in our emergency room that he was in trouble because I had already seen cases like this too many times coming out of the oil field. He had physical evidence for sepsis. He had physical evidence for a stroke. The patient had possible neurologic injuries from head trauma or a stroke; he had an artificial heart valve that most likely was infected; he was a drug user with many more suspected, but unknown, problems.

As Kathy and I were in the process of inserting intravenous and bladder catheters into our semi-responsive patient, the lab technician came in to report that a preliminary stain of the man's blood revealed many blue-stained organisms resembling streptococci and staphylococci bacteria, which are normal germs found on the skin. She set up bacteria cultures with the blood sample and told us that more definitive results would be available in twenty-four to forty-eight hours. This was not good news at all because the staphylococcus bacteria can be extremely dangerous when inside the body. The organism grows in clumps and, in this case, on the man's artificial heart valve and sends out little emboli of infections throughout the body. This becomes particularly troublesome when the infected emboli go to the brain and produce strokes.

About this time one of the EMTs in the emergency room, who had been looking through the man's wallet for identification, called out and said, "Hey Doc. Do you remember this guy?"

I replied that I did not recall him.

His retort was, "Well, his name is Ezra Montgomery, and he's got a DOT card with your name on. His drivers license says he's from San Francisco, California."

Now that he mentioned the circumstances, I told the EMT that I vaguely remembered performing a DOT examination on a large man from San Francisco months before who figured if he could ride a Harley he could drive a truck. I wondered out loud if he ever got that trucking job.

While the pharmacist and the nurse were getting intravenous antibiotics started to combat his infection, I arranged for an air transport to a regional hospital in Billings, Montana. Several hours later we had the man as physically stable as possible, on antibiotics, and on his way via airplane to the regional hospital.

The next day I received separate calls from the regional hospital's neurologist, cardiologist, and infectious disease experts. In total they noted that Mr. Montgomery, unfortunately, had pretty much what I had suspected and reported to them. Indeed, he was septic with staphylococcus in addition to multiple other organisms that had severely damaged his heart valves, including his artificial valve. There were septic emboli that most likely had caused most of his neurologic problems. The best the neurologist could tell at the time was that Mr. Montgomery had incurred at least one stroke and was blind toward his right side; he couldn't tell yet how extensive the damage was. None of the doctors was very optimistic for his long-term prognosis. One of the specialists quipped, "We are throwing as many medical resources as we can at him, but he is still going to die."

A couple days later I received a call from Doctor John Heiser, the heart surgeon at the Billings Clinic, who was always a real gentleman. He told me our mutual patient, Mr. Montgomery, had an angiogram performed by one of the cardiologists that revealed a leaky mitral valve near the suture line. This defect was most likely caused by the staphylococcal infection. Doctor Heiser said he wouldn't attempt to replace the heart valve with a ten-foot scalpel because at the time the mortality rate for that type of replacement procedure approached 100%. However, as always, he thanked me for my kind referral, and he apologized for not being able to help this patient.

Today, replacing an infected heart valve is attempted only in selected cases, especially when the valve fails and the patient has acute heart failure. The mortality rate today is much less than the near 100% quoted by Dr. Heiser in 1979.[37]

The doctors were unable to control the infection in Mr. Montgomery's body or the subsequent hemorrhaging in his brain. An autopsy revealed that infection had eaten away the tissue near the heart valve, which caused it to fail, and the patient died instantly. The pathologist reported that there was evidence of septic emboli throughout the body with literally hundreds of old and new hemorrhages in the brain.

I thought to myself, "All that expense for nothing and the man suffered greatly. Unfortunately, his lifestyle had greatly impacted his health and his poor outcome. It was too bad that Mr. Montgomery did not die at the scene of the accident."

Just A Migraine

Family medicine in a rural or, in my instance, a frontier community is very much like Forest Gump's comment, "Life is like a box of chocolates. You never know what you're going to get." I never knew what kind of medical problem was going to walk through our hospital's doors or what problem an unknown patient would present in the next examination room. That's what made my profession so challenging, yet so rewarding.

One August day in 1977 my clinic nurse Georgia attached a note to a patient's chart and then placed the chart in the basket on the examination room door. The note read, "From out of town and has a migraine. Just wants a shot." The routing slip for charging the patient had a checkmark on the box for NEW PATIENT. Since I had been in Sidney for a short time, most of the patients I saw had this box marked, so this was not unusual. What was unusual was that the patient was already telling me what was wrong with him and knew what the appropriate treatment was.

When I walked into the room I noticed a middle-aged man probably in his sixties who appeared in no acute distress, which was unusual for someone supposedly having a severe migraine attack. I introduced myself, gave the man a handshake, and he introduced himself as Mr. Stanley Whitaker from Minnesota. With a calm voice Mr. Whitaker told me he was having another severe migraine headache. Continuing with the story, Mr. Whitaker said his old family doctor in Minnesota told him his headaches were migraines induced by stress. Periodically Mr. Whitaker received a shot of Demerol, a narcotic medication, for the pain. Mr. Whitaker then handed me a piece of paper with a scribbled notation on a prescription form from the doctor explaining Mr. Whitaker's situation. The prescription looked legitimate to me, but I wasn't convinced that Mr. Whitaker was having a migraine headache because he just didn't appear ill. When I appeared to be thinking a lot about what to do, Mr. Whitaker asked if I could hurry up and give him a shot so he could continue with the family gathering that was occurring at the time. I told Mr. Whitaker I was not in the habit of giving someone I did not know a potent narcotic pain medicine without knowing for sure what was wrong with him. Therefore I told him that I needed to examine him before I would order any medication.

Mr. Whitaker said something like, "Well, if you have to Doc, but make it quick would you?"

Mr. Whitaker told me that indeed he had been having a lot of stress at work before the headaches started. However, he added that the headaches never went away and varied in intensity throughout the day. He related no visual abnormalities with the headaches, nor were they throbbing in nature. He had no difficulty with sensitivity to light called photosensitivity, which is almost a universal symptom with migraine headaches. Nonetheless, he did say that sometimes the headaches would awaken him at night. The Demerol shot usually took the edge off the pain but rarely made him sleep. I knew that none of this man's symptoms matched a history for migraine headaches.

I asked Mr. Whitaker if his family doctor had performed any tests to which he replied that the doctor made the diagnosis over the phone without ever examining him. The small-town doctor knew him and his situation at work so the diagnosis of migraines was a no-brainer. After the patient told me more of his history, I was convinced his headaches were not migraines.

My examination revealed normal vital signs. His head and neck exam revealed a middle-aged man with male pattern baldness. His facial skin was interesting in that half of his face appeared to be oily while the other half was dry. I also noticed that his right pupil was larger than his left pupil. The upper eyelid on the left appeared to be drooping just a little bit compared to the right. Additionally, when I shined a light into his right eye, the pupil constricted briskly and normally. When I performed the same maneuver on the left eye, the pupil reacted slowly. I had not seen this phenomenon before so I excused myself from the examination room to quickly research my findings in a medical school text by DeGowin and DeGowin titled *The Bedside Diagnostic Examination,* a mainstay at my medical school for the bedside diagnosis of common clinical problems. After a few moments of reading I found what I was looking for: Horner's syndrome, a collection of findings associated with a major nerve dysfunction from a lesion in the chest or brain. Now I knew I had to start looking for more things that could cause these additional neurologic findings along with headaches.

I returned to the examination room, apologized to Mr. Whitaker for my interruption, and continued with my examination. While I was palpating his neck for lymph nodes, I asked Mr. Whitaker if he ever smoked cigarettes. He told me he was a two pack a day man since his twenties. I found no enlarged glands on his neck. However, deep palpation behind his clavicles revealed multiple abnormal hard lumps. I found no more enlarged lymph nodes or masses when I examined the armpits, behind the neck, in the abdomen and in the groin areas. My chest examination revealed a decrease in his ability to blow out air, which would not be uncommon for someone who had smoked cigarettes for forty years. Nevertheless, with both inspiration and expiration I heard a whistling noise, or wheezing, in the man's chest on the upper left side. Listening to his heart revealed no obvious extra sounds or abnormal beats. My neurologic examination also revealed a slight weakening of his left arm strength compared to his right despite the fact that he was left-handed. Mr. Whitaker denied noticing any difference in arm strength. Next I had him hold both his arms straight out parallel to the floor with his palms pointing toward the ceiling. I then asked him to close his eyes and keep his arms extended. Within a few seconds the left hand started to rotate inwardly, a forearm motion called pronation. This abnormal neurologic finding is seen when there is muscle spasticity and weakness of the offended arm. The current term for this finding is *pronator drift*, or in my medical school years, it was called the *Barré test* named after a French physician who first described the phenomenon in the early 1900s.

I told Mr. Whitaker that I knew he had headaches and that although he was told they were migraines, I didn't think so. I asked if I could go ahead and obtain x-rays of his head to be sure. Mr. Whitaker looked at his watch and wanted to know how much longer all this was going to take because he had family waiting for his return. I suggested that all of it could be done within the next half hour.

He agreed to the x-rays.

I called Doctor James Garrison, the radiologist at the hospital, and talked to him about my suspicions. I asked him to oversee a full series of x-rays of my patient's head and his chest and to call me as soon as he had interpreted the films.

He agreed.

Since the x-rays took longer than I had anticipated, I was concerned Mr. Whitaker was going to be upset with me because of the delay. When I finally walked into the room to see him again and before I had received the radiology reports from Doctor Garrison, I noticed that Mr. Whitaker appeared different and asked him if he was okay. He said the radiology doctor spoke to him briefly and said he needed to have a long discussion with me.

At just this moment Georgia knocked on the examination room door and said Doctor Garrison was on the phone wanting to talk to me. I excused myself from Mr. Whitaker and told him I would return soon.

On the phone Doctor Garrison told me that my patient was in trouble saying that the man's skull x-rays revealed a shifting of the calcified pineal body, which suggested a mass effect in the brain.

The pineal body is a small pea-sized structure located in the middle of the brain that among other things produces the chemical melatonin, which helps to control wake and sleep cycles.

With age, calcium deposits may be found within the organ. Before the invention of CT scanners and MRI scanners, a calcified pineal gland was one landmark in the brain that radiologists used to help determine if there was a mass effect in the brain. A pineal body shift from its normal position of just one millimeter could indicate a significant brain problem.

Today, high speed CT and MRI scanners with far greater resolution of the brain structures have eliminated the need to search for a calcified pineal body on a standard x-ray. Still, the pineal body shift is an important finding with the newer scanning techniques of the brain.[38,39]

Dr. Garrison told me that if he looked carefully he thought there was a density variation in the right hemisphere of the brain suggesting a mass. In addition, the chest x-ray revealed a mass in the upper portion of the left chest. He took the liberty of performing another series of x-ray tests called tomograms, which essentially took pictures of the lungs in slices. (This was the test used well before the time of the CT scanners.) Doctor Garrison told me, "He's got a big mass in the left main stem bronchus. Looks to me like a big lung cancer." It was his bet the lung cancer had spread to the man's brain and his remaining days were numbered.

I asked Mr. Whitaker if his wife or other family members were available for a group discussion. Mr. Whitaker replied that immediately after he talked with Doctor Garrison, he had called his wife; she was waiting the reception area. I had Georgia escort the wife to the examination room. Two grown children who lived in the area accompanied their mother.

I had the unfortunate duty of explaining to all the family members present that indeed Mr. Whitaker had headaches, but, unfortunately, they were not migraines. I then explained to them my physical findings as well as the x-ray findings of Doctor Garrison and suggested that Mr. Whitaker needed to see his own doctors in Minnesota. I told him I would be glad to send him with the records that we had produced. The family members expressed their gratitude but wondered why his usual doctor treated him for migraines. I could only tell them what I knew.

I told Mr. Whitaker that I was going to give him a prescription for some powerful narcotic pain pills that he could use as he needed so that he wouldn't have to go to doctors' offices anymore to get shots. The family wanted to know how long Mr. Whitaker had to live. I replied that they had asked a God question since only He knew the answer. All I could say was that my patient was very ill and may need more medical care.

The family then inundated me with a lot of questions to most of which I had no answers. Essentially all I could say was that Mr. Whitaker and I had known each other for only a couple hours, and I had determined that he had a very serious medical problem. I encouraged the family to discuss their next course of action among themselves and with his doctor in Minnesota. As they left my office, I gave the family copies of Mr. Whitaker's x-rays along with Dr. Garrison's reports.

Lung cancers have a poor prognosis with an average life expectancy after diagnosis of eighteen or fewer months. Over the years many treatments have been used to treat lung cancers, but none have been very effective. The number of patients surviving five years with treatment is only about ten percent with the least aggressive tumors. The results are much worse for aggressive tumors.

In 2015 a drug named Opdivo (nivolumab) was approved by the FDA (Food and Drug Administration) and highly marketed for the treatment of advanced lung cancer. The contention is that for lung cancer patients with no hope for living longer, Opdivo may allow the patient to live twice as long when compared to treatment with regular chemotherapy that has already failed. The advertisements do not mention that the maximum expected extension of life is only about three months if the treatment works, and the drug produces a tremendous array of serious adverse reactions. The cost for the first three months' of treatment is a mere $141,000. If the patient is fortunate enough to survive and can take the medicine for a year, the drug cost alone is $256,000. When all other treatment-associated costs are added, a year's treatment would cost over $1 million.[40]

Medicare will pay most of the expense. So I ask, "What is a few months' of additional misery worth?" If someone else pays the bill, "It could be priceless."

I never received word of any kind from family members or doctors in Minnesota about Mr. Whitaker. Some of their friends in Sidney, however, told me via the grapevine they had heard Mr. Whitaker went to The Mayo Clinic where he died a few months later while receiving chemotherapy.

Upset Stomach

Essentially all of the harvesting was completed for the year in late autumn of 1978, and the farmers and ranchers were preparing for the coming winter's activity. Harvey, who lived on a ranch about sixty miles west of Sidney, arrived in my office late one afternoon without an appointment complaining of not feeling very good. My nurse Georgia told Harvey that the clinic had been very busy, but she would find a time for him to be seen as soon as possible. She offered the man a seat in the reception area and told him that she would call him soon. Harvey found himself a seat in the packed reception room and awaited the nurse's summons.

When I came out of an examination room, my nurse confronted me and said she had a rancher who drove a long way into town because, "He didn't feel good." Georgia, who was born and raised in the Sidney area, told me that ranchers just don't drive to town because they don't feel good. She figured Harvey must be pretty sick, told me the man looked awful, and wanted me to see him next. Georgia knew far more about our clientele than I, and her judgment in these matters was excellent.

Georgia escorted Harvey to an examination room while I went to my office to dictate a note on my last patient's visit. Entering the examination room, I saw a man perhaps in his forties who appeared ill, but not acutely so. After we shook hands and exchanged introductions, I started to query Harvey about his concerns. He started to tell me that he had had an upset stomach all day that would not go away. He related his history of ulcers and treatment for years with diet and antacids prescribed by Dr. Johnson who had moved from Sidney the previous fall.

Before he could say another word, Harvey vomited a large dark blood clot about the size of a nine-inch emesis basin onto the floor. This was followed almost immediately by another emesis of bright red blood. Having been in this situation several times before, I knew that I had an acute medical emergency on my hands.

I opened the examination room door and yelled for Georgia to bring a wheelchair STAT! Upon her arrival, I loaded Harvey into the chair, and as I was wheeling him out the door to go across the parking lot to the hospital, I asked Georgia to notify the hospital emergency room of my situation and that I was on my way. Before I got out the door, Georgia told me that she would advise the other patients in the reception room of an emergency and the office staff would do their best to reschedule the patients for another day.

Harvey vomited once again as we were racing across the parking lot to the emergency room where the charge nurse and the lab tech met us at the door. Before Harvey knew it he was on an examination table with two intravenous lines in his arms. The laboratory technician obtained blood for testing and a crossmatch of stored blood for a possible transfusion, the surgery team was alerted, and the new general surgeon in town, Dr. Rogers, was summoned on an "I need you right now" basis. Our team soon determined that Harvey was anemic and his blood pressure was low. I knew that we needed to stabilize him soon with blood and a lot of intravenous fluids and that he needed surgery immediately.

In his short time in Sidney, the hospital staff had learned that Dr. Rogers wasn't comfortable caring for acute emergency surgery cases because of potential litigation. Indeed, over the next half hour or so, Harvey continued to vomit blood and I was having difficulty maintaining his blood pressure with blood and fluids alone. I had to convince Dr. Rogers that the man needed an immediate operation to stop the bleeding. Reluctantly, he agreed, and we took Harvey to the operating room on an emergent basis. As she was about to put Harvey to sleep, the anesthetist forewarned the surgeon and me that our patient might wiggle when the skin incision was made but assured us that Harvey would not remember a thing. She cautioned that she was doing her best to increase our patient's blood pressure, but the anesthetics tended to lower blood pressure even more.

After we got Harvey prepared for the operation, the anesthetist gave him some anesthetics and placed a breathing tube into his throat so he would not aspirate blood into his lungs. Dr. Rogers made an incision in the upper middle abdomen, and yes, Harvey did wiggle a bit. When the abdomen was opened, we immediately visualized the stomach distended with blood. Dr. Rogers made a hole in the stomach to drain the blood and to find a source of the bleeding. The stomach had some raw ulcerations, but we saw nothing that was actively bleeding. We then searched in the area just past the stomach called the duodenum and found a good-sized artery actively pumping bright red blood. Dr. Rogers ligated the artery with several stitches and all the bleeding stopped. We decided to wait just a few minutes to allow the anesthetist time to stabilize our patient with blood and fluids, and she did. As we were cleaning out the abdomen and closing all the holes that we had made, making sure again that all the bleeding had stopped, Dr. Rogers noted that the man would require a partial gastrectomy in the near future to prevent further episodes like this. A partial gastrectomy was a common surgery at the time for recurrent ulcer disease during which part of the stomach was removed and reattached to the small intestine.

Harvey tolerated this emergency procedure well and during his subsequent hospital stay displayed no obvious ill effects from the surgery or the eight units of blood that he received to keep him alive. Before he left the hospital I had a discussion with Harvey regarding the possibility of a surgery if his symptoms recurred.

I did not see Harvey for another six months after this episode. For whatever reason, he decided to visit my office for a follow-up checkup before he started spring planting. Since his surgery, Harvey reported that he had religiously continued with the same antacids and special diet that had been prescribed to him some years before by Dr. Johnson.

In January 1979, a new drug came onto the market named Tagamet that inhibited stomach acid secretion. The drug had been tested and sold in England for over a decade before it came to the United States,[41] and I attended a symposium about the new drug about a month before Harvey's appointment. I told him about the new medication and suggested that he give it a try. I even had samples to give him for a month so the drug was not going to cost him a penny. Harvey agreed to try the Tagamet. Before leaving my office I advised him to stop his antacids and special diet once he started taking the pills. Harvey was agreeable to the idea but was a little doubtful. Nonetheless, he was desperate to eat a steak again. The rest, as we say, became history. Harvey never had another problem with his stomach.

Tagamet, its generic name is cimetidine, worked so well that it became the original blockbuster drug by having yearly sales over $1 billion. The drug was so effective that the partial gastrectomy surgery, which was one of the more common surgeries performed by general surgeons at the time, essentially vanished. The drug spawned a revolution in ulcer management.

Only four years later in 1983, Barry Marshall, an internal medicine physician from Perth, Australia, discovered that a spiral bacterium named Helicobacter pylori was associated with most stomach ulcers. Additionally, it became apparent that the bacteria also caused stomach cancer.[42] Dr. Marshall's discovery along with the development of acid blockers like Tagamet were monumental steps in medicine that changed suffering ulcer patients from having marginally effective palliative treatments to receiving opportunities for cures.

It took a decade or more for doctors to accept Marshall's discovery. It seemed that doctors had difficulty imagining a little bug like Helicobacter pylori causing so much trouble. (Have you ever seen an engine sputter with just a small piece of dirt in the carburetor?) Today doctors test ulcer patients routinely for the bacterium and treat those infected with large doses of antibiotics. Interestingly, the bacterium often returns to the stomach after treatment yet does not cause ulcers again. We do not know why.

In 1996 I tested Harvey for the Helicobacter pylori bacterium, even though he was doing well on his Tagamet medication. As I suspected the test was positive. I offered antibiotic treatment to kill the germ to diminish his risk for stomach cancer, and my patient had already been on Tagamet almost continuously for seventeen years. My patient had suffered no adverse effects from the Tagamet, had experienced no further episodes of bleeding, and was now over sixty years old. Harvey was a commonsense kind of guy and a rancher. He said he was doing fine and if it wasn't broke, don't fix it! Nonetheless, he offered to think about my offer.

A Special Man

Robert McRae was born in a farmhouse during the early days of the Great Depression and just at the beginning of the great American drought, or the Dust Bowl. His parents were sheepherders in central Montana. Robert spent the first few years of his life living with his parents and siblings in a sheepherder's wagon in the remote hills and high plains of eastern Montana. Before he was a teenager his father died, and Robert became the man of the house for his three younger siblings and his mother. He was forced to grow up well before his time.

While in high school, Robert spent some time with the local doctor in Jordan, Montana, and soon developed a desire to become a physician and help his mentor in rural Montana. After graduating from High School in Jordan, Montana, between the end of World War II and the beginning of the Korean War, Robert continued his education at the University of Montana. During these years that he discovered mathematics and physics, and Robert soon dropped all thoughts of being a rural doctor to pursue a career in science. After graduation Robert entered the army as a second lieutenant just at the end of the Korean conflict. Unlike many of the unlucky men of his age group, he did not have to participate in the Korean War only to become another wartime casualty statistic.

Soon after graduation Robert married his college sweetheart and together they started a family and he started his career in education. By the mid 1960s Robert had earned a PhD from the University of Wisconsin and took the meaning of his doctorate degree to heart (The word doctor is derived from a Latin word meaning teacher) by continuing to pursue a distinguished career in education at Eastern Montana College, which was later renamed Montana State University Billings. Initially teaching physics Dr. McRae advanced to the chairman of the college's sciences department and finally rose to the position of Dean of Graduate Studies and Research. Along the way his expertise in solving physics problems garnered him considerable national recognition as an expert in accident reconstruction. Indeed, Robert McRae was a very smart and talented man.

Dr. McRae was my boss in college where I worked as a teaching assistant in the physics department for three years. During our many discussions I learned about Dr. McRae's past, and he learned about mine. Since we both came from financially challenged families, we had a lot in common. When I received my Doctor of Medicine degree, Dr. McRae was one of the first to call to congratulate me. Over the passing years we remained in contact; I was in my medical practice in eastern Montana, and he was advancing through the educational ranks at Eastern Montana College.

One day during my sophomore year in college while I was preparing a room for the next physics laboratory session, I noticed Dr. McRae sitting at his desk and crying. When I asked if there was something I could do, he told me he had just had a frightening, but exhilarating, experience while he was walking from his home a few blocks away to the science building. Without further provocation he started telling me a story about one of his foster children who had gotten into trouble. He and his wife Beverly were struggling to decide whether or not they should cancel their efforts with this child and stop caring for foster children altogether. Dr. McRae noted that their foster son, an Indian boy, had made him very angry by getting into trouble with the police. Visibly moved by the experience, which was unusual for the normally sedate Dr. McRae, he said that as he was walking along the irrigation canal toward the school, "Someone spoke to me." He said he looked around and no one was there. As he continued walking, he heard the voice again. Turning around and looking in all directions, all he saw was a bright light in the sky. The voice was coming from the bright light. He knew he had experienced a revelation, but just didn't know what it was. Dr. McRae told me that he was a man of science and always expected there had to be something else. Now he had a good idea.

Over the coming years Dr. McRae and his wife Beverly would accept almost twenty foster children, adopting many of them. He became comfortable in his new role as a scientist and a man of faith. He did not necessarily believe in a God according to some religious book, but he did believe in a universal force. Dr. McRae and I had multiple talks during which he relived his experience by the irrigation ditch.

After I completed my first book, *Reflections of a Country Doctor* about experiences as a rural family physician, I presented Dr. McRae with one of the first copies. Now in his early seventies, he told me that he couldn't remember squat for any length of time. He could still do his physics calculations using a slide rule and mathematics, but he couldn't remember what he had for breakfast ten minutes before. He asked me if he had Alzheimer's disease because he was still the primary caregiver for his wife. She had suffered a stroke a few years before that had impaired her speech and thinking. He was concerned he might make a mistake that could hurt his wife.

I told Dr. McRae everything I knew about Alzheimer's disease and finished by letting him know that in general these patients are forgetful, but they don't care about not remembering things. He was forgetful and he did care. Therefore I did not think his forgetfulness was of the Alzheimer's type. I suggested some medical texts he could read and gave him the names of several neurology doctors in the area he could consult to learn more about dementia, and particularly Alzheimer's disease.

Alzheimer's disease is named after a German physician named Aloysius Alzheimer who in the early 1900s observed a middle-aged female patient with profound short-term memory loss along with other interesting behaviors for over five years. After her death his team examined her brain tissue using special staining techniques developed by one of his colleagues. They found what would become the diagnostic pathology findings in the brain for this type of premature dementia.

Unfortunately, even today using sophisticated testing procedures and imaging techniques, the absolute diagnosis of Alzheimer's disease can be made only after an autopsy of the patient's brain. The disease remains a curiosity because its etiology is uncertain, and its clinical course is variable in duration and severity. Since the early 1990s several types of drugs have been promoted to treat Alzheimer's dementia. Unfortunately, the drugs have not significantly modified the natural conclusion of the disease.[43,44] Today we know much more about Alzheimer's dementia than did Dr. Alzheimer and his colleagues in 1906. However, the diagnosis is still made mostly by clinical observation and no curative treatment exists.

When I published a second book, *The Next Prescription*, I gave Dr. McRae a copy. He showed me the medical texts and all the articles he had obtained from the college library to learn as much as he could about the different types of dementia and Alzheimer's disease. After critically reviewing the scientific studies, he concluded that the treatments didn't work. I agreed with him.[45,46]

By now I noticed that he could still carry on an adequate conversation, but he kept forgetting things in the middle of a sentence, and when he would catch himself repeating things, he became annoyed. Yet he was still able to function adequately to care for his wife in their home. It was during this meeting that Dr. McRae once again tearfully relived his revelatory experience on the ditch bank with me; he told me that he had finally figured out his conundrum during all his years in science: there must be balance, there must always be balance. He went on to explain that he had always dealt with the four known dimensions of science problems: length, width, depth, and time. Now he knew there was the fifth dimension called the human spirit. He then went on to tell me that there was so much evil in the world that many more individuals had to perform good deeds to make things balance out. He figured during all those years of helping kids he and his wife had done their share to maintain the balance in nature.

When his wife died about a year later, Dr. McRae's mental status deteriorated relatively quickly. I do not know if his progressive dementia was Alzheimer's disease or something else. I believe Dr. McRae lost all interest in life after his beloved wife died, and he really died in the nursing home of a broken heart.

I will forever be grateful for our wonderful conversations during my college years and beyond. A kind man and a wonderful mentor ... Robert McRae, PhD

A Rocky Adventure

I was awakened in the early hours of a Friday morning by severe pain in my back and in the middle of my abdomen on the right side. After I got out of bed and walked around our home, the discomfort abated somewhat for about ten minutes. The pain then returned with a vengeance and now included severe discomfort going into my right genital area associated with vomiting. Soon the vomiting just became retching into a toilet bowl with nothing coming out. Ten years before I had an episode with a kidney stone on my left side. That kidney stone got stuck and required surgical removal. I thought that now I might be passing another kidney stone.

To complicate my presentation, I had recently undergone a hernia repair on my right lower abdomen and the greatest share of the discomfort in my abdomen was directly over the surgical scar. I wondered if somehow I had torn apart my surgical repair. Over the next several hours the pain would come and go along with the nausea and retching. Finally after I had no relief with the severe pain and nausea for three hours or so, I awakened my wife to take me to the hospital emergency department.

To my amazement the discomfort intensified during the ten-minute trip to the hospital so that by the time we arrived at the hospital I had difficulty getting out of the car. Before walking into the emergency room I had to stop on the sidewalk because I was bent over with pain. Once inside I bent over with discomfort twice before I was able to make the short walk to the reception desk. The woman at the reception desk could see that I was having difficulties and asked if I needed a wheelchair. When I asked how much farther I had to go, she pointed to a room perhaps thirty feet away. I told her I thought I could make it; I barely got there before I doubled over with pain and had to sit down again.

A nurse's aide was summoned to assist me and she supported me into the room. After I gave her my name and birth date, the nurse assistant was able to locate my file on the hospital's computer. As I was giving her a brief history of my problem, and I do mean a brief history, the woman obtained my vital signs using an automated machine. I recall that she was having difficulty getting the machine to work properly because I kept interrupting her with my retching into the now ever present vomit bag. Back in the day we used reusable kidney shaped containers or buckets, but now the disposable containers resembled inverted plastic sorcerer's hats. Soon an emergency department nurse arrived, introduced herself, noticed that I was a physician, saw that I was in considerable distress, and wanted me to tell her the level of my pain between zero and ten. Knowing how I must have presented myself, I stared at her and asked if she was kidding. Quite professionally she repeated her request, and I replied that I was going to give my pain a ten.

Within a few minutes I was taken by wheelchair to an examination room where the nurse helped me onto an examination table, repeated my vital signs, obtained a little more history, and told me that the doctor would be in to see me soon. Before she left, the nurse asked about my pain level. I told her it had not changed. Apparently the nursing staff and the doctors were required to ask every patient about their pain status every visit. It seemed irrational in my situation because the medical team knew I should not receive any pain medicine until a diagnosis was made.

Perhaps ten minutes later a young emergency department physician entered my room, looked at the computer screen, and again took the same brief history of my current problem. After a short examination of my abdomen and back, he told me the radiology department was going to get a CT scan of my abdomen to see if they could find out what was going on acutely. Before the doctor exited the examination room and knowing that I was a physician, he asked what I thought I might have. I told him I had narrowed my self-diagnoses down to four things: (1) a kidney stone, (2) damage to my recent right inguinal hernia repair, (3) acute appendicitis, or (4) any combination of the three. The doctor promised we would find the answer pretty soon.

Before the doctor got out the door I started to have dry heaving again so he said he would request some medicine to relieve the nausea. He also told me that he was going to have the lab come to draw some blood for testing and have the nurse come in to start an IV to give me some fluids.

I thanked him for his efforts.

A lab technician came first to obtain some of my blood for testing. The nurse followed soon thereafter and inserted an intravenous catheter into my arm and hooked it to a bag of fluid. Within a short time a young woman from the x-ray department took me to obtain a CT scan of my abdomen. Oddly enough, this radiology technician used to live in Sidney; I delivered her as a baby.

Fortunately, the latest versions of the CT scanners are very fast because she had to take a picture of my body between my episodes of retching. I remember the days when our hospital in Sidney, Montana, got its first CT scanner, how slow it was in taking pictures, and how I had to restrain patients even for simple scans so they would not move. A good scan of the head would take about half an hour or more. The new scanners took seconds.

After the scan was completed I was transported back to my examination room where the nurse was waiting for me with two syringes, one medication for nausea and another medication for pain. Perhaps ten minutes later the nurse returned to ask me about my pain number. I replied my ten score was perhaps a nine and one half. The nurse responded she would get something more for pain and left the room.

I found that having a lot of pain made time pass incredibly slowly while I could only look at the ceiling in the examination room. However, what seemed hours to me in waiting was probably only a short time before the doctor came in and told me I was correct on at least one of my diagnoses, a kidney stone.[47] He told me the stone appeared to be quite small and should pass. Therefore, he said I could go home, encouraged me to drink a lot of fluids, and wait for the darn thing to pass. As always, if I got worse or if I developed a fever, he asked me to return. As a precaution, he gave me a prescription for some pain pills, which was curious because I was still nauseous and intermittently having dry heaves. Kay took me home to obey the young doctor's orders.

By the time we got home, I was feeling a lot better. I thought to myself that perhaps the stone did move down into my bladder, and I was done with it. Fortunately, the nausea and pain medicines from the emergency department had started to work; I was feeling pretty darn good. I consumed water like crazy and subsequently spent most of the day going to the bathroom. Unfortunately I did not pass a stone. I remained relatively free of discomfort for the remainder of the day and went to bed that evening with no nausea, no fevers, and no pain.

Early in the morning I was again awakened with right-sided pain that unbelievably was exponentially worse than the day before. The vomiting was followed by dry heaves and then the retching started. This time I developed sweats and chills, so once more Kay returned me to the emergency department at the hospital. Again I had to stop several times before I got to the reception desk. The clerk at the reception desk, who was different from the day before, asked me the same questions. The nursing assistant and the emergency department nurse also were different from the day before. This time, however, when one of the nursing personnel asked me to give her my pain score between zero and ten, I muttered, "37!"

I went through an evaluation process similar to the previous day only this time I was told my kidney functions were off the charts, the kidney stone hadn't moved, and my right kidney was swollen from the backup pressure, a condition called hydronephrosis or swollen kidney. The emergency room doctor summoned the urology surgeon on call who apparently was performing a surgery in the hospital up the street several blocks away. Subsequently, I was admitted to a hospital bed to await the urologist's visit and the surgical removal of the stone obstructing my right kidney. In the meantime I was to be given copious amounts of intravenous fluids, anti-nausea medications, and intravenous pain medicines to keep me comfortable. Multiple nursing personnel admonished me not to put anything in my mouth before surgery. I thought to myself, "This is a bit of a no-brainer since I had been vomiting and retching for almost twelve hours."

The urologist came to see me later that morning, advised me that she had had multiple emergency surgeries to do that morning, and that I would be advised by the nursing personnel when it was my turn. In the meantime, she was hopeful that the nurses could keep me comfortable with medication and make sure I was well hydrated before surgery. I knew this meant a lot of intravenous fluids and more trips to the toilet.

When the time came Kay and I were escorted to the preoperative staging area outside the operating rooms. It was the weekend and the surgery team was short staffed; only a single nursing assistant was available to watch over me. We had been told that I would be going right into surgery. After waiting a considerable amount of time in the preoperative area, one of the personnel came to inform us that the urologist had encountered a complication during her procedure, and I would have to wait a little bit. By now, the pain medication and the anti-nausea medication had worn off, and amazingly, the pain in my right back became even worse then it had been so far. Again I started retching into the vomit bag. Kay summoned the nursing assistant to see if she could help me. The young woman came to my bedside, saw me dry heaving into the vomit bag, and naïvely asked, "Are you nauseous?" With my face stuck into the vomit bag and looking at this woman, I thought to myself, "Duh, what do you think?"

Apparently realizing that she was in a situation beyond her pay grade, the young woman left to try to find someone who could help. A few minutes later a woman dressed in a surgical scrub suit came through the surgical doors, saw me gagging into the vomit bag, and told us she would talk with the anesthesiologist. She then walked quickly back into surgery. Soon thereafter someone else returned with syringes filled with medicines to help my nausea and pain. Perhaps half an hour later my pain was slightly improved, my nausea had improved, and I was wheeled into surgery on a gurney.

The next thing I remember was that I was waking up in my room. I did not know what time it was, but I could see that it was dark outside. I knew I wasn't throwing up but I still had an excruciating, unremitting pain in my right mid back and similar pain in my right groin. My right testicle felt as if had been hit with a hammer. While I was still groggy from the anesthesia I recall a nurse coming to my bedside and asking me to rate my pain from zero to ten. I do not recall what I told the nurse except that the pain in my back was really bad. Soon she returned and gave me more medication through my intravenous line and said she would be back soon to see how well it worked. When she returned, and I don't recall the timeframe, I reported to her that the medication did not seem to do anything. She told me she would call the doctor, and they could try something else. After several more attempts to control my pain, the nurse gave me something that worked. All I could think was "Thank goodness."

I was up most of the night going to the bathroom and collecting every drop of bloody urine in the appropriate container by the toilet, and there was a lot of it. The urologist had placed a stent, a small, long flexible straw, in my right kidney and ureter (the tube from the kidney to the bladder) to allow my right kidney to drain all the extra fluid and blood it had accumulated, and it drained all night. Every time I got up to go to bathroom I developed severe pain in my right back followed by nausea and dry heaves. I guessed this situation was as close as a man could experience what a woman experiences in early pregnancy with morning sickness.

I remembered my grandpa William Schmockel who everyone called Smokey. Grandpa was born in the 1890s and had watched the development of the automobile in America. He would often tell us that Henry Ford's Model T or Tin Lizzie was a wonderful machine, and to keep them running, the name said it all. FORD stood for Fix Or Repair Daily. I was beginning to feel like a model T that required fixing or repairing daily.

The following morning the urologist came to visit and reported that my right kidney was pretty beat up. She noted that she had performed an x-ray using dye once her catheter got into my kidney. Because of the amount of blood and swelling that were present, she wanted to see what she was dealing with. The pictures revealed leakage from the backside of my kidney. I knew when she said this that I was not in a good situation. Blood and urine are meant to stay where they're supposed to be in the body. The human body does not like extra blood and urine floating around on the inside, and it responds appropriately with a severe inflammation. The gist of what I recall from her comments was that (1) there's blood and urine on the backside of my right kidney, (2) the kidney stone was still in my right kidney, (3) the decompression stent in my right ureter was to remain for two weeks to allow my kidney to heal, and (4) I had to return for another operation to retrieve the kidney stone. Later that day I went home in misery.

The next two weeks were pretty much like the movie *Groundhog Day*. That is, everything seemed the same. Whenever I lay down to rest per doctor's orders and got up, the severe pain in my right back migrated to my right lower abdomen and my right testicle. Nausea and occasional vomiting returned too. I could only describe the feeling in my back as two pieces of Velcro fiber ripping apart when I stood up and then reattaching after a few minutes. Actually, after I thought about this for a bit, the sensations made perfect sense. Whenever someone stands up the kidneys normally drop a short distance because of gravity. Therefore, whenever I lay down, the right kidney returned to its normal position. Whenever I stood up, the right kidney dropped just a bit, which was normal, but in the process it tore apart the adhesions they were part of the healing process on the backside of the kidney.

After two weeks I returned to the outpatient surgical center to get the stent and the stone out. All I recall being told by the urologist after the surgery was that the stone, which was only three millimeters in size, was removed, I had a congenitally small right ureter which trapped the very small stone, and if I ever had another kidney stone I should tell the surgeon to remove it promptly. Finally I had another stent inserted that needed to be removed at home in ten days. The little relief from back pain I had afterward was much appreciated. Kay then took me home again to rest.

The positional pain in my back and right side remained. This discomfort would eventually persist for more than a year. On the assigned day Kay removed the stent that was draining my right kidney. Despite some localized discomfort, I felt a lot better because the stent had been causing a lot of bladder spasms that made me urinate frequently. When I went to bed that evening I felt pretty good. Unbelievably, the next morning I was again awakened with severe pain in my right back going into my right lower abdomen and into my groin associated with the return of nausea and vomiting. Following the urologist's post-operative instructions, Kay took me to the emergency room for third time. Repeat CT scans revealed a swollen right kidney again, and my kidney functions had dramatically deteriorated again. This time I was admitted promptly to the hospital.

When the urologist saw me in my hospital room she told me that there were no more stones but the entire right kidney and ureter essentially were swollen shut. She admitted that she had not seen this situation before. Her other colleagues in the urology department had not seen the situation before either. Collectively the urology team saw no benefit with my undergoing another procedure to put in another stent. The stent would just cause more swelling and it would be another do over. Hence, the urology team decided the best course of action was benign neglect. I thought this was a pretty good idea because I didn't want to undergo another operation. The course of treatment included narcotic analgesics for pain, medicine for nausea, anti-inflammatory drugs, such as ibuprofen, to decrease the tissue swelling, and close observation.

A middle-aged physician came into my room not long after the urologist's visit. He introduced himself as the hospitalist, and he was responsible for my care while I was in the hospital.[48] Before he had a chance to take my history or to perform an examination, his pager went off; he said he had a sick patient elsewhere and had to go. The doctor returned the next day in the afternoon, asked a few questions about my medical practice in a frontier zone, looked at the computer monitor, and left. The third day he came in to say goodbye. He said his physician assistant would make my discharge arrangements even though my urologist had done this earlier. In three hospital visits this specialist in hospital care never took my history, never touched me, and finally pawned off the paperwork, or computer work, to a subordinate. He did, however, charge for a comprehensive admission examination and three days of acute care. My first experience with hospitalist care was bad.

With my course of treatment I slowly felt better over a few days. At least I improved.

Over the next six weeks the nausea resolved. However, the right back discomfort radiating to the right lower abdomen remained. When I returned to the young urologist's office for a post-operative evaluation, my minimal activity of that morning was enough to produce severe pain in my back and right lower abdomen. When the urologist evaluated me, she was again perplexed. She noted that nothing she did should have caused discomfort in the right lower abdomen, and the crack in the kidney should be well heeled after six weeks. The doctor had a medical student with her at the time, and I allowed the student to examine me. The urologist stepped out of the examination room to consult the clinic's chief of surgery and arranged for me to see him right away.

By the time I saw the surgeon, my pain was once again almost unbearable. After an examination, he thought I might have a trapped nerve in the scars from my recent inguinal hernia repair that worsened by all the swelling from my recent adventures with a small kidney stone. He subsequently made an appointment for me to see an anesthesiologist that day for a nerve block procedure that I had a couple hours later. The anesthesiologist, guided by an ultrasound picture, fortunately was able to locate the correct nerve and injected it with a local anesthetic. When he stabbed the nerve, which he really didn't mean to do, I had a shooting pain into my right groin; but when he injected the local anesthetic, the acute pain was gone almost immediately. Interestingly, and I told this to the anesthesiologist, the pain in my back went away too. Needless to say this was unexpected and the doctor was just as befuddled as I. However, I wasn't going to complain about the additional benefit. If I had only known to get rid of my back pain I needed a shot in my groin, I would have had them do it weeks before.

The right back and groin pain did return, but to tolerable levels. After some thought and some reviewing of my medical school anatomy texts, I determined that the blood and urine that leaked out of the back of my kidney inflamed the two significant nerves that cross over the lower one-third of the kidney. These nerves provide sensation to the groin areas, and they were obviously injured somehow. I had developed a chronic pain syndrome. As I mentioned earlier, the pain in my right back and right groin would continue for another year until I had another medical adventure, and I would learn to appreciate Grandpa Smokey's FORD analogy. I just hoped I didn't need to be fixed or repaired daily.

I performed an Internet search seeking a statistical analysis combining all the probabilities for the adverse events that happened to me just because a tiny three-millimeter kidney stone got stuck. One in two million was the result. I knew my urologist had worked a lot with statistics before entering medical practice, so I made her a card that stated all my complications and ended with, "The probability of all these things happening to a single patient was one in two million. Your removal of my three millimeter stone...PRICELESS!"

A Bug Story

In medical school in the early 1970s I was taught that a natural breakdown in the body's immune system as we aged caused cancers. Children and young adults who developed cancers were assumed to have some undetermined immune defect. As a medical student working in a family planning clinic in Portland, Oregon, in 1973, an attending physician, who was a gynecologist with a private medical practice, presented to me a young woman patient having her first female examination and already had cervical cancer. At the time he taught me that sometimes bad things just happen because most cases of cervical and uterine cancer were found in older women and were the result of aged-related immune system changes.

The idea that an infection with microscopic organisms could possibly be the culprit in cancer was heresy, not because there was any proof against the idea, but because nobody had looked to see if there was any association. Still, when reputable scientists made excellent observations and correlations about health and disease, the medical establishment often discarded them.

Mentioned somewhat in passing, our microbiology professors noted that an Italian physician named Rigoni Stern in the 1830s observed that celibate women, especially nuns and Jewish virgins, almost never had cervical cancer whereas prostitutes frequently had the disease. These observations suggested that female genital cancers were possibly sexually transmitted diseases. These observations occurred thirty years before Louis Pasteur promoted his germ theory of disease in the 1860s, and they went virtually unnoticed for another one hundred fifty years.

An example to demonstrate an individual's influence on medical thinking in the 1800s is the story of Dr. William Mayo speaking at the American Medical Association in 1894. The distinguished speaker of the day was the surgeon general of the army who presented a paper on the increasing incidence of cancer in eastern America. The fundamental point of his paper was that cancer was increasing in the United States and evidence suggested that it might be an infectious disease.

Dr. William Mayo from Rochester, Minnesota, was in attendance and after dissenting intensely with the surgeon general's assertion that cancer could be an infectious process assumed the podium. Dr. Mayo later recalled his remarks and spoke to this effect:

"I am from Minnesota. It seems to me that this is the way it is. Cancer is preeminently a disease of 40 and beyond. Only the young people who were in good enough health to struggle with the development of a new country came to Minnesota from the East, leaving the people of cancer age behind. There was therefore greater freedom from cancer in the new state. Now Minnesota is older. The young people are moving on, leaving behind a larger percentage of people in the cancer age, and we noted an increase in cases of cancer just has happened in New England and the older states. As to the old houses, they're more likely to be inhabited by old people of cancer age. And anyway the question of coincidence must play a part. I'm not a poker player, but I am told that a perfectly honest man can sometimes hold four aces."[49]

The conclusion afterward was that cancers are obviously a disease of the aging process and not from an infection. These kinds of comments made from merely observations or experiences by influential leaders in the medical field became dogma for almost the entire twentieth century. This concept of cancer is the one I was taught in the 1970s.

At a meeting I attended in the mid 1980s, I learned that a doctor named Harald zur Hausen in Germany proved that a common virus was associated with cervical cancer. Since then it has become clear that the virus is involved somehow with many cases of cervical cancer, and there is little doubt in the western medical

community that preventing this viral infection could all but eliminate cervical cancer in women worldwide. In fact, a vaccine is
now recommended in America for young teenagers to prevent
this viral infection and hopefully eliminate female genital cancers. Unfortunately, some who have received the vaccine have
developed female genital cancers, so the concept has flaws. As a
biologist at heart the vaccine idea seemed to me to be another
attempt to have a single simple solution to a most complex problem.

Near the turn of the century when asked about microbes
causing cancers, Anthony Fauci, MD, the Director at the U.S.
National Institutes of Health said, "There have been many, and
there will be more, for when you look, you find. Fifteen years
ago," he notes, "most doctors doubted that viruses played any
role in cancer; now the consensus is that they cause around
twenty percent of cases. And it will turn out to be a lot more than
that."[50]

Dr. Paul Ewald from Amherst College noted, "Evolutionary
theory leads me to conclude that sexually transmitted pathogens
cause a lot more problems than we are yet aware of. They must
survive a long time in the host, hidden from the immune system;
the only ones that survive will have figured out that trick."[51]

While working for over three decades attending female
patients in family planning clinics, public health clinics, and my
private clinic I evaluated and treated many women with abnormal tissue on their uterine cervix that was found by a Papanico-
laou test or PAP test. Back in my early days the tests were
reported as either normal or graded for abnormal cells by mild,
moderate, severe, or cancerous distinctions. In the late 1980s
pathologists developed a more detailed and specific grading system according for the PAP test by what would be called the
Bethesda system or TBS. The name came from the location of the
conference, Bethesda, Maryland. Along with the new grading
system came updated guidelines for the evaluation and treatment of abnormal cells on the cervix.

By 2000, the evidence for cervix abnormalities being a venereal disease associated with a certain type of virus was mounting. The newer treatment options zeroed in on removing virus-infected cells. All too often, however, the treatment was unsuccessful and the virus returned, or a patient developed cervical or uterine cancer without the virus being detected. In 2004 at a family planning clinic I attended a middle-aged virgin with cervical cancer whose initial PAP test at age forty-five was cancerous, and no evidence for the virus was found. Certainly her cancer was not sexually transmitted and perhaps not caused by the suspected virus. This not uncommon case history produces a definite dilemma for the infection-and-cancer-connection theorists.

So now by 2015 medical thought surrounding microbes and cancer has made a full circle; it only took about two hundred years. From Rigoni Stern's observations in 1832 to Pasteur in the 1860s promoting the germ theories to Dr. Mayo and others' condemning observations about germs causing disease to Dr. Fauci at the National Institute of Health in the twenty-first century admitting that germs are indeed a major component, and in fact, the cause of many chronic diseases and cancers. However, germs are not and cannot be the singular answers.

Could it be that the disruptions we have produced in our body's bacterial populations by using and abusing antimicrobial drugs during the last half century are associated somehow with the new epidemics we now face such as AIDS, asthma, SARS, obesity, mental illness, diabetes, attention-deficit disorders and cancers?[52] Certainly, no simple answers exist and only time and careful study will reveal the true importance of germs and disease processes.

A Matter of Fat

When inadequate oxygen is delivered to the heart muscle, the muscle may be damaged. In medical terms this is called ischemic heart disease. There are probably many reasons for this process to occur, but the most common cause of ischemic heart disease is thought to be a process called atherosclerosis during which sequential layers of a cholesterol rich plaque material is deposited inside the arteries of the body. The coronary arteries are the blood vessels that carry oxygen-rich blood to the heart.

The known associated risk factors for the development of ischemic heart disease are many and among others things include a strong family history for heart disease, advanced age, tobacco use, poor physical conditioning, high blood pressure, elevated blood fats, and others.[53]

Prior to the 1950s the medical profession made few inroads into treating ischemic heart disease. Since nothing could be done about someone with a strong family history for heart disease, which was considered to be responsible for up to seventy percent of cardiac risk at the time, marginal efforts were made to change a patients' modifiable risk factors for heart disease.

Atherosclerosis, or hardening of the arteries, begins early in life depending upon each person's physiology and for reasons that are uncertain. After the Korean War a study was published in the 1950s containing the results of autopsies performed on soldiers killed as a result the war which revealed that even though the average age of the dead was just over twenty-two years, there was noticeable evidence of coronary atherosclerosis in a varying degrees in seventy-seven percent of the autopsies, and three percent of the soldiers had at least one heart vessel totally occluded.[54] To be sure, these men were not the athletic, physically fit specimens of today's volunteer army, but they were recruits from the general population nonetheless, and these soldiers were young men with significant heart disease. The findings from this report energized the medical, biochemical, and pharmaceutical professions to pursue answers to how and why cholesterol-laden plaques filled arteries. Cholesterol in the blood was deemed to be the primary culprit, and the amount of effort to find a cholesterol modifying solution was enormous. Consideration of addressing other modifiable risk factors for heart disease fell to the wayside. Doctors and patients wanted and started looking for an easy answer to a complex problem.

Then along came Akira Endo, PhD, a Japanese botanist who admired Alexander Fleming, the Scottish botanist credited with discovering the antibiotic penicillin from mold. As a young scientist in Japan Doctor Endo's work centered on the use of natural fungal enzymes in the processing of fruit juice. He made multiple successful discoveries in this endeavor for which he gained considerable recognition and was granted a sabbatical at Albert Einstein College of medicine in the mid 1960s as a research associate working on human cholesterol.[55]

In this work he discovered that many fungi produce chemicals that allow them to ward off parasites by inhibiting the parasites' ability to make their own type of plant cholesterol, a necessary building block for the plant's cell structure. Subsequently, he and others determined that fungi produced an internal chemical that was similar to plant cholesterol and inhibited the parasite's production of cholesterol. This chemical event prevented growth of the fungi's parasites.

Dr. Endo studied thousand of compounds and found three from a certain mold that inhibited an enzyme necessary for cholesterol production. In the mid 1970s, one these chemicals named Mevastatin (also named compostin) became the first in a new class of chemicals called statins that were shown to lower blood cholesterol levels in humans.

Starting in 1987 many anti-lipid drugs became commercially available with the presumption that lowering blood cholesterol levels would automatically equate to less ischemic heart disease.

The doctors, patients, and drug companies wanted a major weapon against heart disease, and they knew it was the statin drugs. This was a presumption and a hope without any proof.

Fantastic claims of reduced mortality rates from heart attacks of thirty percent or more from supposedly unbiased studies sent the medical community into a tizzy. Doctors knew they had a reliable weapon against cholesterol, considered to be the #1 modifiable risk factor for ischemic heart disease, and some supposed experts predicted that heart attacks would soon become a medical curiosity. The drugs were marketed aggressively, and I actually had a pharmaceutical representative try to convince me that his drug would *decrease death* by thirty percent. I informed the man that everyone dies and that death, as far as I knew, had been one hundred percent since the beginning of time.

Within a decade the statins became the best selling class of medicines in history. There was little doubt these medications decreased the levels of all the types of fat compounds in the blood, and there were multiple studies purporting the effectiveness of these drugs in decreasing mortality rates for all people with heart disease. At least, that's how the drugs were marketed.

On closer scrutiny, however, the studies revealed that indeed the drugs were effective in only slightly improving the mortality rates for a very small group of individuals with a history of previous heart attacks. For patients over sixty who did not have heart disease, the studies showed the drugs had no benefit. Additionally, there was no benefit ever shown for any woman of any age who took the drugs. According to Dr. James Wright, a professor at University of British Columbia and director of the British Columbia Therapeutics Initiative, "Most people are taking something with no chance of a benefit and a considerable risk of harm."

Comments like these caused an uproar in the medical community. For years the populace had been bombarded with the message from doctors, hospitals, the media, and pharmaceutical companies that high cholesterol levels must be brought down because blood cholesterol was everyone's ticket to an early grave, and the statins were the major weapon against high cholesterol. Some researchers even suggested, hopefully jokingly, that everyone should be taking statin drugs and perhaps municipalities should put them in the drinking water just like fluoride.

Printed advertisements for Lipitor, the statin drug with the largest market share, proclaimed, "Lipitor reduces the risk of heart attack by thirty-six percent...in patients with multiple risk factors for heart disease." With these results, how could any reasonable physician or patient resist taking these drugs when they claim to reduce your mortality rate by thirty-six percent?

These statements came into question when the results of a major study called ENHANCE were released in January 2008. The study revealed that the statin drugs, even when several drugs were given together to lower lipid levels further, had no benefit on heart attacks and deaths from heart attacks.[56,57]

Close review of Pfizer's printed advertisements for Lipitor reveals an asterisk beside the thirty-six percent figure. In very small type the official language of the report is, "...that means in a large clinical study, three percent of patients taking a sugar pill or placebo had a heart attack compared to two percent of patients taking Lipitor." Simply stated, the evidence revealed that only one person out of a hundred patients had any measurable effect from the drug. Or, vice versa, ninety-nine percent of people had no benefit. The drugs do lower blood levels of cholesterol, but that alone did not reduce or eliminate heart attacks. The drugs were never shown to improve the incidence of, or the deaths from, heart attacks and they never did. The published results were all statistical manipulations and marketing ploys. Indeed, another big lie.

Statins have been sold now for over thirty years. To date, the expected dramatic decreases in morbidity or mortality from ischemic heart disease have not occurred. Unfortunately, a significant increase in the number of severe adverse effects from the statin drugs have emerged, especially in patients over sixty:

memory loss, decreased ability to think, muscle pains, peripheral neurologic problems, and many others.

I met an acquaintance in the fall of 2015 as I was writing this piece for the book. He's a seventy-year-old man whom I will call Arnie. Arnie was aware that I was a physician and cornered me just to tell me his story. The fellow explained that he had had a stroke about six months before, but now he was doing okay. He elaborated by demonstrating to me which parts of his body did not work then and worked now. To my surprise his extremities appeared to be working almost normally when I saw him. Arnie told me in great detail how he went through rehabilitation for many months to enable him to walk again.

After seeing how well he was doing, I told Arnie I was impressed at his progress since I saw him golfing that day.

Arnie continued to report that his stroke specialist told him that the reason he had a stroke was because the cholesterol in his blood was too high. The doctor then gave Arnie a statin drug to reduce his cholesterol. Becoming angry, Arnie told me that within three days of taking that medicine he couldn't walk again. His neighbor told him to look up the medicine on the internet, which he did. Arnie then asked me, "Do you know what I found?"

I knew what Arnie probably found on the internet, but I didn't say a word. I just let him talk because it was apparent that he needed to vent to somebody.

Arnie told me he found that the drug he was prescribed wasn't worth a damn in people over sixty-five. For sure it wasn't any good for people who had strokes. But it did cause muscle pains and weakness, which he had. Arnie then went on to tell me that his neighbor was a nurse at the same hospital stroke unit and told him to get off of those medicines before they killed him. The nurse directed him to another neighbor who gave him a diet and exercises to help reduce his cholesterol. Arnie told me he hadn't had a piece of steak, a piece of sausage, or a hot dog for over four months, his cholesterol level had come down a few points after three months, and he thought maybe he felt better.

As he was leaving, Arnie wanted to know why the stroke doctor gave him those medicines that might kill him when he knew they weren't any good.

I could only wish Arnie good luck with keeping his cholesterol down, but I told him I thought it would be all right if he had a hamburger once in a while.

Despite the information available to doctors, the statins remain the largest selling class of drugs.

A Colossal Lie

Early one fall morning in the mid 1990s I received a call from our emergency room. The nurse said, "Doctor A, I need you now." When I asked about the problem, the nurse replied, "Just come." Having received similar calls over the years, I knew not to question the nurse and to just go to the hospital. After I arrived the ER nurse told me she had a woman visiting from out of town with really painful breasts. I was perplexed since sore breasts did not seem to me to be an acute emergency, and besides, I was not on call. The nurse escorted me to see the patient.

Forty-five-year-old Elaine Norris was sobbing and told me she was awakened by excruciating pain in both of her breasts. She said they became hot and hard suddenly as if she had just stopped breast-feeding. Unfortunately, her youngest child was now eighteen years old and a senior in high school. Elaine had always been a healthy, athletic woman who had only seen a physician for her three pregnancies and routine examinations. She had never been seriously ill, but now she was worried something was dreadfully wrong.

My exam revealed a woman in considerable distress. She was sitting on the exam table with the gown open in front exposing her breasts because she said the pressure from the cloth was too painful to bear. Her breasts were red, hot to touch, swollen, and exquisitely tender to my minimal touch. She was afebrile, and except for enlarged lymph glands under her arms, her examination was unremarkable. Except for a breastfeeding woman with mastitis, I had not seen breasts in this condition.

I asked the nurse to give the woman enough morphine until she was comfortable. Also I asked the nurse to apply gauze pads soaked in ice water to the breasts in an attempt to relieve some swelling. I had no idea if this would work, but I figured t was worth a try. In the meantime I went to the medical library to research the causes of acute breast inflammation and concluded that Elaine must have acute inflammatory breast cancer. Unfortunately, the definitive diagnosis required a breast biopsy after the acute swelling had resolved. If I was correct, this woman had a very bad problem because, as I garnered from my reading, this type of cancer usually has spread in the body when it is diagnosed.

After several doses of morphine numbed her acute pain, Elaine wanted to know what was happening. I told her that her breasts became inflamed for some reason, and a biopsy would be needed to find the exact cause. I offered to give her enough pain medication to last until she could visit with a physician in her hometown. Her husband agreed with my plan and said they would travel home as soon as they left our emergency room. Elaine thanked me for the pain medicine and the cool wraps on her breasts. Because of the time of day the local pharmacies were still closed. Therefore I had the nurse obtain enough narcotic pain pills from the hospital's pharmacy to last for several days and make copies of our ER records for our patient's doctors. Elaine left our ER with less pain, but obviously not well.

I now step back fifty years to my high school days in 1965.

Every morning Fred Kayser dressed for work as a high school physics teacher in Billings, Montana, with a dark suit and a bright bowtie. When he arrived in his classroom and before he addressed his first physics class of the morning, Mr. Kayser took a clean eraser and cleaned the blackboard. He then retrieved a clean cloth from the supply closet and wiped out the loose powder in the chalk tray below the chalkboard. Finally, he carefully placed one piece of white chalk in his white chalk holder and another piece of yellow chalk in his yellow chalk holder. He then waited patiently at his neatly organized desk for his students to arrive.

Not only was Mr. Kayser meticulous with his attire but also with the way he taught physics to senior high school students. Each time he wrote on the chalkboard, he apologized to the class for not facing them. After he used the chalk, he would wipe his hands with a clean cloth. After lunch, which he called the noon meal, Mr. Kayser performed the same ritual with the chalk and the chalkboard trays that he had done in the morning. Never did I see a speck of chalk on his black suit; he left work in the afternoon just as clean as he came in the morning.

One day while my lab group was performing an experiment, we became confused because we were not getting the results that we anticipated. Mr. Kayser came by to check our progress, and our group members explained about our getting unexpected results. He dutifully looked at our calculations and told us that the observations and the calculations we had made were correct. The facts were the facts. Mr. Kayser pointed out that facts represented what was true, not what we wanted them to be. Our facts did not match our hypothesis. Therefore, our job was to explain the facts that we had obtained instead of trying to manipulate our calculations into something we thought they should be. He reminded us that, "Science was about being accurate and being truthful, not about being wishful."

In college my various science professors promoted the same concept; that is, science requires careful and accurate observations along with truthful recordings of those observations. There was no place in science for dishonesty. During my college years while I was working as a teaching assistant I promoted this scientific mandate of careful observations and meticulous honest recording of the findings. Facts were facts, and it was our job to figure out what the facts meant.

Effectiveness and Efficiency was a book written by an English physician named Archibald Cochrane in 1971.[58] Dr. Cochrane's book criticized medicine for using interventions and treatments without any reliable evidence for their effectiveness. His demands for more systematic reviews in medicine eventually were instrumental in laying the foundation for what we now call "evidence-based medicine," a concept that physicians should treat patients with therapies that have proven effectiveness through appropriate unbiased clinical testing. The idea was simple: make sure the treatment works before you use it. In essence, physicians should follow the Hippocratic oath, and foremost they should knowingly do no harm to their patients.

Upon graduating from medical school, Robert Bacon, PhD, my advisor and well-respected scientist in anatomy, encouraged me to continue with my scientific thought process after I got into medical practice because medicine is forever changing. He cautioned, "Believe nothing you hear and only half of what you see," and "Remember that half of what you learned in school won't be true in five years."

In 1992, I was a physician member of the Board of Directors of Blue Cross Blue Shield of Montana when a woman with metastatic breast cancer petitioned Blue Cross and Blue Shield of Montana to pay for a bone marrow transplant. Her oncologist had told her that a bone marrow transplant was the only way for her to survive, and at the time, our company did not pay for such experimental procedures. Therefore, her request for payment was denied. This denial set into motion a sequence of legal issues that our board discussed at length. Throughout the discussions at the board level, the doctors insisted that a bone marrow transplant for breast cancer was an experimental procedure while the lawyers insisted that there was documentation in the medical literature that validated the effectiveness of the treatment. In time Blue Cross and Blue Shield of Montana felt compelled to pay for this woman's treatment.

Indeed, there were articles in the medical literature that purported the effectiveness of a bone marrow transplant given after chemotherapy for advanced breast cancer failed. Alternatively, however, there were skeptics among the oncology profession who noted that no accredited clinical trials had been performed. Unfortunately enthusiastic reports such as the one in December

1989, in the Washington Post reported that the Johns Hopkins University had found some "partial success" with bone marrow transplantation for breast cancer. This article also noted that the treatment would cost between $75,000 and $100,000 and "is usually covered by health insurance or Medicaid." Unfortunately, the statements were untrue. The Johns Hopkins data were speculation within a very small sample of patients, the procedure was known to be experimental, and as a rule, health insurance companies did not pay for experimental procedures.

In 1990, a cancer physician in Maryland told a thirty-five-year-old mother of three children that her "best chance of surviving more than a year" was a bone marrow transplant, which her insurance company would not pay the cost. The woman subsequently sued the insurance company and a federal judge ruled in her favor stating: "To require that the plaintiff or other plan members to wait until somebody chooses to present statistical proof … that would satisfy all the experts means that plan members would be doomed to receive medical procedures that are not state-of-the-art." Less than a month later a federal judge in Massachusetts ordered another insurer to pay for a bone marrow transplant for another woman with metastatic breast cancer. Without any evidence to the contrary that they were willing to consider, the media had a heyday with these story. The health insurance industry was vilified, the legal system was canonized, and the dying patients received the high tech, expensive health care they wanted.

The writing was on the wall. Judges had determined that they knew what was best and made medical judgments for the populace. Insurers were mandated to pay for bone marrow transplants for dying women with metastatic breast cancer, even if the procedure did not work.

In late 1990, the Blue Cross and Blue Shield Association of America, knowing that they would eventually be ordered to pay for the expensive experimental procedure, offered to invest in a national clinical trial including women with metastatic breast cancer. This was the first time a private insurer had agreed to fund a trial of treatment. Certainly, this decision was a response to the emotional nature and controversy regarding breast cancer and potential lawsuits.

In 1994, the office of personnel management ordered all health plans serving federal employees to grant coverage for bone marrow transplantation to women with breast cancer within twenty-four hours or risk being dropped from the federal program. Near the same time, the National Cancer Institute argued there was too much scientific uncertainty about the effectiveness of transplantation. No one listened to the National Cancer Institute experts.

In 1995, the Journal *of Clinical Oncology* reported a second promising study again from South Africa regarding bone marrow transplantation in women with metastatic breast cancer. The article was widely hailed as proof of the effectiveness of the procedure. Bone marrow transplant centers started up all over the country, and insurance companies were forced to pay the astronomical costs.

Four years later in 1999 at the annual meeting of the American Society of Clinical Oncology, five studies were presented regarding bone marrow transplantation in women with metastatic breast cancer. The South African investigator reported impressive results again that equaled his previous papers. Interestingly, the four other major studies revealed no improvement in outcomes.

Several months thereafter, auditors from the United States and Europe journeyed to South Africa to validate the claims of the clinical trials and found total fabrication.[59,60,61] In 2000, the South African investigator admitted that he falsified his results and relinquished his position at his university. Incidentally, it was determined that the doctor had essentially made up scientific studies for over twenty years.[62] The breast cancer bone marrow transplant programs mostly in America had been built based upon a lie.

After this revelation, the health insurance companies again declined payments for the procedures. The government did not complain, and the lawsuits stopped. The lawyers and their clients who had won lawsuits under false pretenses did not give any money back. Insurance companies eventually paid over six billion dollars for about thirty thousand women to suffer through this procedure. An estimated fifteen percent of the women died prematurely from the treatment.

Sometime later I learned that Elaine did indeed have inflammatory breast cancer and underwent chemotherapy, bilateral mastectomies, and radiation therapy. The cancer was not halted, and she continued with a bone marrow transplant procedure. After the transplantation was completed, Elaine was perpetually sick. She experienced horrific adverse effects from the anti-rejection drugs she was required to take as well as from the medications given to minimize the effects of the other drugs. In addition, despite the transplant, the breast cancer continued to eat away at her body. Just before Christmas Day in 1997 Elaine declined further treatment and died peacefully at home with her family. She became one of the statistics of women who died prematurely from the bone marrow transplant procedure.

The lifeblood of the medical profession is scientific research. This includes research for drugs, orthopedic devices, high-tech treatments for cancers, and many others. Our patients trust us, their doctors, because their lives and wellness may depend upon us. In turn, we doctors must trust the information we receive from our colleagues performing scientific research. When presented with scientific data, we must be able to accept that data at their face value because we believe our colleagues are honest. We always have a right to disagree with the interpretation of the facts or how a particular research study was performed, but preserving confidence in one's colleagues is essential. Trust has been and must be the basis for scientific endeavors to endure and for doctor-patient relationships to remain viable. The South African doctor admittedly lied to his fellow physicians around the world who in turn subjected many women to a devastating course of treatment that did not work.

As Mr. Kayser emphasized to his students fifty years before, "Science was about being accurate and being truthful, not about being wishful."

An Aging World

Over the years I was asked to discuss many topics in medicine. When asked about what I thought were the biggest changes in medicine that I had seen, I often talked about the effects of non-medicine on health and the problems we face with managing an aging population. Having experience as a nursing home medical director and geriatric educator for many years, I became acutely familiar with many of these issues. This presentation has been modified and updated over the years, but the facts and the principles are the same.

In September 1970, an elderly senior professor was making introductory remarks to our freshman class orientation as the University of Oregon Medical School class of 1974. He told us that he considered medicine his calling and hoped that someday we would feel the same way. The doctor mentioned that during his lifetime the life expectancy in America had increased from about forty-five years of age in 1900 to approximately seventy-one years in 1970. He emphasized that this statistic alone was proof of the wonders of medicine. After the professor finished his introductory speech, our class started our studies.

During the second year of medical school, our class had a six-week course with Dr. Harold Osterud, the chairman of the Department of Public Health and a local medical historian. Dr. Osterud was important in the medical curriculum, at least to me, because he talked about the history of medicine. He discussed relevant statistics and how to interpret them in medicine as well as population dynamics, which was my biology major in college. Possibly most important to me, Dr. Osterud tried to get our class thinking about what the treatments in medicine today might have on future populations.

Dr. Osterud cautioned that from a public health standpoint, "Medicine has not been as productive as your other professors have made it seem." He pointed out the comments made at our orientation regarding the improvements in life expectancy in the past seventy years. He explained that life expectancy numbers are nothing more than mathematical calculations that start when you were born and have little correlation with the lifespan, or the maximum life attainable, of a population. He continued to inform the class that information from the 1700s showed the habitants of colonial America to be healthier and wealthier than their counterparts in Western Europe. The anticipated life expectancy at birth in 1700 in America at thirty-five years was longer than the British at the same time. The life expectancy at birth of the English population at the same time was only twenty-eight years. Dr. Osterud then reminded us that the life expectancy calculation from 1900 given to us during our orientation was just forty-five years, a mere ten year improvement in two centuries. [63,64,65]

He wanted us to appreciate the difference between life expectancy at a certain age and lifespan, the actual lifetime of a population. In humans, the lifespan was considered to be about 120 years. He noted that if thirty-five years was the maximum lifespan in colonial times, then there would have been few to attend the Continental Congress since only a couple of the delegates were older than thirty-five years. In fact, Benjamin Franklin was in his seventies. John Adams was in his early forties and did not die until 1826 at the age of ninety. Thomas Jefferson was thirty-three years old in 1776. George Washington was in his mid-forties. This illustration points out that the life expectancy at birth is a calculation, not a fact. The life expectancy calculation for 1700 requires other input including the number of children who died early, the number of women that died with childbirth, the number of people who died prematurely from frequent outbreaks of infectious disease such as cholera, infectious diarrheas, diphtheria, smallpox, typhus, typhoid fever, and malaria. The population of colonial America had to deal with the public heath issues of fouled water supplies, absence of sanitation, and other assorted maladies especially in the urban areas. Dr. Osterud added that if an individual survived all of these bodily insults during colonial times, he or she would have lived a long time, as did Benjamin Franklin, Thomas Jefferson, and John Adams.

After this discussion, Dr. Osterud analyzed the information given to our class during our orientation that because of the wonders of medicine, the life expectancy in America between 1900 and 1970 increased by twenty-six years, He emphatically pointed out that the statement was not true and was not caused by medicine. Being a medical historian, Dr. Osterud pointed out that the germ theory was discovered in the mid 1800s and promoted by Louis Pasteur who was a microbiologist and a chemist, not a physician. The implementation of the germ theory and the eradication of bacterial contaminations by:

(1)   Developing and building sewer systems and water treatment facilities by civil engineers,

(2)   By teaching people to wash their hands and to bathe more frequently with soap and water, and

(3)   By teaching the people through books, newspapers, and social interactions to cook food adequately, to boil water, and to eat better made a significant difference in overall nutrition, infant mortality, maternal mortality, and many infectious problems.

The results from these simple measures, which had nothing to do with doctors or medicine, were that the mortality rate went from forty per 1000 people in 1700 to only fifteen per 1000 in 1910. This large reduction in mortality rate resulted from dramatic decreases in infant and maternal mortality. At the same time the life expectancy calculation at birth in 1910 increased almost forty percent to forty-eight years. Interestingly, Dr. Osterud recognized that if a person survived to sixty-five years in 1910, his life expectancy increased to almost eighty years and noted the similarity to longevity in 1700 if the person survived the early life bodily insults of the era.

The mortality rates continued to drop for several generations until antibiotics were discovered and made available for general use by the medical community in the 1950s. By 1970 the mortality rate in United States dropped further to about seven per 1000 population, while the life expectancy at birth calculation had increased to about seventy years.

Dr. Osterud asserted, and wanted us to appreciate, that the population data showed about an eighty percent reduction in mortality rates and a near doubling of the life expectancy at birth calculation without any significant intervention by the medical community. He emphasized this point again hoping we would remember that the health of a population is not a simple matter and is based upon a lot more than the work of physicians, hospitals, and the medical community. Dr. Osterud pointed out that the life expectancies of all populations around the world, even in the poorest of countries, was increasing without the wonders of medicine.

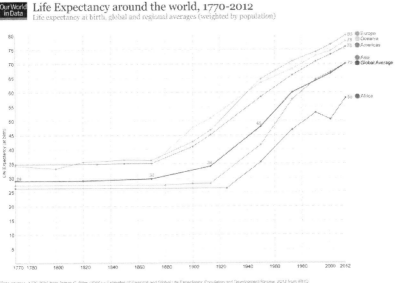

Life Expectancy around the world, 1770-2012
Life expectancy at birth, global and regional averages (weighted by population)

After a short pause in thought, Dr. Osterud reflected that the phrase, "Cleanliness is next to godliness," has merit for longevity worldwide.

Concluding his remarks, Dr. Osterud stated that, "I hope the purpose of your wanting to be doctors is to help people live better and longer. But always remember we have to look at the Public Health side of the coin. What happens if we become too good at helping people, the population lives too long, and normal population dynamics get all messed up?" He then challenged us with, "Imagine what the expense could be to society if people get too old? Let's hope we can make people live longer and better."

Because of the way my medical training was structured, I spent most of the next three years concerned about whether or not my hospital patient would live until the next day, or whether or not my intensive care patient would live until the next hour. I spent no time thinking about the consequences of prolonging older patients' lives suggested by Dr. Osterud.

In 1965, the legislation to enact Medicare and Medicaid as part of President Lyndon Johnson's "Great Society" was passed by Congress. The law, which was a supplement to the Social Security Act, entitled the elderly and the indigent to healthcare services regardless of their income or previous health status. Prior to this act, the elderly and the chronically ill paid substantially higher health insurance premiums than those who were young and healthy. Additionally, the act mandated that hospitals, if they accepted any government payments, had to accept and care for all patients despite their ability to pay. Additionally, the act mandated desegregation of all medical care services, medical care providers' offices, and hospitals if any government payments were received. This bill also included nursing home payments on a limited basis. The law became active in 1966, and the demands for services by the elderly and the poor overwhelmed the system. In time, however, various parts of the medical care system expanded their services attempting, quite unsuccessfully, to meet the growing demands of Medicare and Medicaid patients.[66]

During my internship in the spring of 1975, I spent some time with a gastroenterologist in Spokane, Washington, named Wayne Atwood. Dr. Atwood was a most caring individual who had a very busy practice of medicine. Normally, he would have eight to ten patients in the hospital with gastrointestinal illnesses. Medicare paid for his elderly patients' hospital care. One day while making hospital rounds, Dr. Atwood seemed to be frustrated with the system of medicine that was evolving because of Medicare and Medicaid, and we sat down to chat about how things were in the real world of medicine, the world that I would be entering soon when I would have my own private practice. Dr. Atwood suggested to me, "If only the government could legislate a Fountain of Youth that we doctors could prescribe and save our patients all their suffering."

On this particular day, Dr. Atwood was having trouble finding a nursing home willing to take an indigent senior citizen patient who had both Medicare and Medicaid insurance. I learned that there were not nearly enough nursing home beds to fill the needs of his patients alone. Additionally, many of his patients really did not need a nursing home. Unfortunately, however, Medicare and Medicaid did not pay for home care services, and a nursing home was the only place to care for his patients after hospitalization if they had no family support. Nursing home placement was not an ideal situation.

As the years passed, and while I was in private practice, the life expectancy at birth gradually increased to over eighty years. The Medicare and Medicaid programs changed continuously adding more services and more eligible people to the programs. Along the way, the government added hospice benefits, dialysis benefits for end stage kidney disease, and home health services for many medical services and diagnoses.

When affordable insurance became available, senior citizens flocked to doctors' offices and emergency rooms in droves. Knowing that they would receive compensation for their efforts, hospitals, local health departments, and private companies promptly developed competing programs to provide services to sick and dying patients. The cost to the Medicare and Medicaid programs, and eventually to the taxpayer, increased astronomically and far in excess of the amounts allowed, or even anticipated, when the programs were enacted in 1965. And still there were more patients demanding care. Health care in America had been transformed from a privilege to a right of American citizenship.

To supply manpower for the increasing need for services demanded by the populace, the federal government, in its wisdom, decreased the funding for medical education. The obvious physician and healthcare worker shortages escalated. A scandal in the Veterans Administration Hospitals in 2013 graphically exposed the divide between the governments' vacant promises for healthcare availability and the reality of failing to provide care to veterans.

In 1965, the House Ways and Means Committee estimated that the hospital insurance program of Medicare, the federal health care program for the elderly and disabled, would cost $9 billion by 1990. In 1967, the House Ways and Means Committee re-projected the entire Medicare program would cost $12 billion by 1990. The actual cost in 1990 was $98 billion.

In 2010, Medicare provided health insurance to forty-eight million Americans—forty million people age sixty-five and older and eight million younger people with disabilities. In 2010 the cost was $182.7 billion, or over 47% of the total cost of hospital care in America. By 2014, the Medicare bill rose to $505 billion.

In 1987, Congress projected that Medicaid, the joint federal-state health care program for the poor, would make special relief payments to hospitals under $1 billion in 1992. The actual cost: $17 billion. By 2014 the cost for Medicaid exceeded $492 billion. The total cost of all health care services in America in 2014 exceeded $4 trillion.[67,68,69]

"Modern medicine was just coming into acceptance in the 1950s and 1960s," said Josh Gordon, a health care specialist at the nonpartisan Concord Coalition, which advocates balanced

federal budgets. "The future advances of medical sciences, and
their inevitably high costs, were not fully appreciated in 1965,"
he said. The mere existence of Medicare helped to raise its long-
term costs beyond projections, Mr. Gordon said. "Medicare led to
increasing life expectancy, which obviously impacted Medicare's
costs as older and older seniors used more and more of its services over longer and longer periods of time."[70]

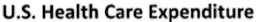

U.S. Health Care Expenditure

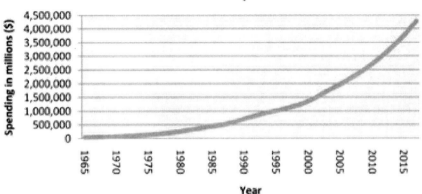

Between 1990 and 2010 there were marginal decreases in mortality rates for all age groups. For example, infant mortality
decreased from nine per thousand (0.9%) to 7 per thousand (0.70%).
Compare these numbers to those between 1700 and 1910 when the
infant mortality rates dropped from up to 400 per thousand (40%) to
about 150 per thousand (15%). During the period from 2000 to 2014,
any statistically significant increase in longevity in people over sixty
years resulted primarily from cardiovascular interventions while
the mortality rates for cancers and strokes remained relatively stable. Some may argue that outcomes for cancers and strokes were
greatly improved. Facts are facts. The presentation of facts depends
upon how one manipulates the numbers.[71]

By 2014, the life expectancy of a child born in America that
year had reached eighty-one years, and the infant mortality had
dropped to an all-time recorded low of 0.65%. To reach this mile-
stone, regrettably, Americans spent at least twice as much as

any other nation in the world. Unfortunately, other nations such as Japan and Sweden, had reached this goal years earlier for a fraction of the cost.

Dr. Osterud died in 2004. I wonder what he told his students in his later years about the costs to our country with our aging population.

Electricity in the Air

Patients brought containers of all shapes and sizes into my office on a regular basis. Usually, my nurse or I had given the patient a sterile container at a previous encounter with instructions to insert a particular type of bodily sample into it, label it, and return it to the office. However, at least monthly, someone brought in a container with something unknown. Often, the patient brought in the sample to help me make a diagnosis. The unknown material usually was a sample of fecal material or something they found floating in the toilet. Foul-smelling, discolored urine was a common entry for diagnosis. Most of the time either my nurse or I would dutifully examine the material and give the patient our best guess about its importance to that person's health.

An elderly man from North Dakota named Jasper brought in my most memorable sample. In passing, Jasper mentioned to me that he had worked in construction as an electrician for over forty years. Jasper handed me a one-quart mason jar with a small amount of brownish liquid in the bottom. The jar lid was screwed on tightly and sealed with black plastic electrical tape. Jasper told me that he had been passing some pretty foul wind lately and figured he must have something wrong inside his gut. At the insistence of his wife, he decided to bring a sample of his foul wind for diagnosis.

I asked Jasper what was in the canning jar.

He told me that he placed the open jar next to his butt and gave it a good electrical fart. He quickly closed the jar and sealed it tightly to preserve the smell.

When I asked Jasper what an electrical fart was, he told me that they are the ones that come out with a little bit of juice. He then looked at me, smiled, and reminded me that he was an electrician.

Knowing that whatever goes into the front end of the bowel determines what comes out, I asked Jasper if he had changed his eating habits recently. He told me there was a new pizza restaurant in Sidney that served a mean spicy sausage and jalapeno pepper pizza. He enjoyed eating cold pizza, so he bought the extra-large size pizza and had some everyday at home.

I wondered to myself, "What should I do with this jar?" I certainly was not going to open it and stink up the whole office. I asked Jasper to sit in the reception area until I examined his electrical fart sample.

Looking through the side of the clear glass jar I saw pieces of undigested material I convinced myself were pieces of jalapeno peppers. I discarded the jar without opening it.

I had my nurse escort Jasper back into an examination room where I told him that there was nothing seriously wrong with him at this time regarding his bowels. However, to keep peace with his wife and his coworkers, I suggested that he cut back on his special pizza to just one day a week.

Reluctantly, he admitted that he suspected I would tell them just that.

Worms

As I entered the examination room I saw two-year-old Brandi and her mother Jessica waiting patiently. As soon as I greeted them, Brandi yelled out, "Dr. Jimmie, mommy brought in the bugs she pulled out of my butt!" Jessica brought with her a small brown paper bag containing a small glass container. When she removed the container from the bag and handed it to me, I could see several worms about three inches long in the bottom. When I asked Jessica how long her daughter had been having these worms, she said for about a month or so. Jessica told me that she was embarrassed because only dirty people got worms, and her daughter took a bath every night. She found some of the worms in the bathtub during the bath. I reassured mother Jessica that having worms had nothing to do with being unclean.

I saw several creatures in the container that looked like common roundworms, also known as ascaris worms. A relative of the human roundworm is strictly found in pigs. Since the family lived in town and I knew they were not raising pigs, I inquired if Brandi had been playing on a farm recently. Jessica told me that they went to her husband's family farm often. However, Jessica noted that the farm had not raised pigs for years.

I informed Jessica that the eggs from the pig roundworm could remain dormant in the ground for years. Therefore, I guessed that Brandi had been playing in dirt contaminated with pig feces and put some of the dirt in her mouth. Consequently, some eggs got into her daughter's intestine where they liked to live and grow.

It was obvious to me that Brandi was not seriously ill from the infestation, which is a common finding with worms in small children. Usually the intestinal parasite causes few if any symptoms in adults and older children.

I informed Jessica that after a few days of taking a certain kind of medicine her daughter should be fine. At this point, Brandi started to chant, "Doctor Jimmie fixed my butt. Doctor Jimmie fixed my butt." She continued with the chant while I was writing her mother a prescription. As they were leaving my office and much to her mother's dismay, Brandi made sure my nurse, my office staff, and the patients in the reception room all knew that, "Doctor Jimmie fixed my buuutt."

As I requested, Jessica brought in a sample of her child's stool several weeks later. The laboratory technician examined the specimen and found no evidence for worms or worm eggs. When I gave Jessica the good results, she was relieved. Now she could stop explaining to people why her daughter kept singing, "Doctor Jimmie fixed my buuutt. Doctor Jimmie fixed my buuutt."

Peanut and Potato

On a spring day in 1980 I had the opportunity to visit for the first time with an exuberant young woman in her twenties named Annabelle and her husband Bradley. They had recently performed a pregnancy test that was positive and were ecstatic about the possibility of becoming new parents. During the visit the couple chose me to provide prenatal care for Annabelle. Over the next few months during regular prenatal examinations, it became apparent that Annabelle's abdomen was growing much faster than one would expect for a routine pregnancy. When she was about twenty weeks pregnant, I distinguished two separate and distinct heart tones. For her first try, Annabelle was having twins!

My training in obstetrics allowed first-time pregnant women to attempt delivery of twins. Unfortunately, it became common practice for obstetricians to jumpstart the delivery process by performing an elective cesarean section before labor started thinking that multiple gestation pregnancies presented too high a risk for the mother and the babies. Unfortunately, this approach led to many C-sections that extracted babies that were premature and required significant management afterward in the newborn nursery. Contrary to the current thinking of the time, I thought that Mother Nature had been performing vaginal deliveries in humans for many thousands of years before surgery was even invented. As a result, I usually took a wait and see attitude to allow mothers to go into labor on their own. Then I knew with reasonable certainty that it was time for the babies to be born.

As the summer progressed into fall and Annabelle's abdomen became massive, I knew she was uncomfortable. However, she never stopped smiling and seldom complained. Always trying to be considerate of others, Annabelle entered the hospital in labor on a Saturday in late September.   Soon after she entered the hospital, it became apparent to me that Annabelle was going to have difficulty delivering her babies naturally. Therefore, I performed a cesarean section to deliver her two babies.

The operation was uneventful. After extracting the babies, I noticed that the infants were both female, but one was substantially larger than the other. Even though they seemed to be identical twins, one of the babies received more nutrition from a larger part of mom's placenta. This was not an unusual finding, and I knew it was not a reason for concern. After the operation had been completed, I had the opportunity to evaluate the babies. Usually with a multiple birth, the infants are labeled by the birth order, such as baby A and baby B or baby #1 and baby #2. Because of the discrepancy in size of these babies, I decided to name them Peanut and Potato. Peanut's birth weight was less than 5 1/2 pounds. Potato's weight, on the other hand, was closer to 7 pounds. The parents gave the girls official names of Allison and Ashley, but for the next eighteen years that I cared for them in Sidney to me the girls remained Peanut and Potato.

Over the years, the parents brought the girls to my office for all sorts of things including routine well baby exams, frequent upper respiratory illnesses and ear infections, and during the junior high and high school years, pimples and sports injuries. Since the family lived in a small town with few students in this school system, the twins participated in many school activities and played every girls' sport. When they weren't participating in a sport, they were part of the cheerleading squad or band. Academically they were superb.

It was the fall of her freshman year in high school when Ashley, or Potato, developed headaches all of a sudden with significant discomfort in her neck. Initially, I thought headaches were thought to be either stress headaches or migraines. Despite using simple measures at home such as local heat, stretching exercises, massage, and anti-inflammatory medications, the headaches did not resolve.

During the next week several things happened to Ashley. First, she had a viral illness with sweats, chills, vomiting, and body aches for which she went to the emergency room and was given intravenous fluids by the doctor on call. Second, she noted that ibuprofen made her headache go away sometimes. Third, during a basketball game she suffered a head injury, which may have been a concussion, and she continued to play the game. Fourth, Ashley developed double vision and put up with the problem for several days before coming to see me.

When I examined Ashley in my office a week after the previous visit, her headache had resolved. However, she definitely had double vision because her left eye was wandering aimlessly while trying to focus. My preliminary diagnosis for this finding was a possible acute sixth cranial nerve palsy of her left eye. I promptly called the ophthalmologist fifty miles away in Williston, North Dakota, and arranged for Ashley to be seen promptly the next morning.

The ophthalmologist called me the next afternoon to inform me that indeed my patient had a sixth nerve palsy that was associated with swelling of the optic disc. He had performed an MRI scan of her head that was read as normal. He suggested that I contact a neurologist or neurosurgeon for consultation, which I did. The neurologist, after receiving my history of the recent events regarding Ashley, noted that the clinical presentation had no recognizable pattern that she knew. With her test being otherwise normal, the neurologist suggested that I perform a lumbar puncture to determine the pressure and appearance of Ashley's spinal fluid. Ashley's mother telephoned me about this time, I passed on the comments of the neurologist, and we made arrangements for Ashley to have a spinal tap procedure performed in our emergency room when they arrived back in town.

I performed the spinal tap on Ashley and recorded her initial spinal fluid pressure as over 500 mm. The normal value would have been less than 200. After I removed a certain amount of clear fluid for analysis, the pressure dropped to near 220, and

Ashley noted that her vision was a lot better. After I consulted the neurologist again with the test results, which were all normal, she recommended a series of medications for my patient to start taking.

While I was waiting for Ashley to complete her observation time after the tests, and while I was waiting for a woman in labor, I reviewed Ashley's medications. Sometime during this interval Ashley's mother informed me that her daughter had been started on a tetracycline medication for her facial acne about six weeks before the headache started. After my research, I concluded tentatively that Ashley's problem might be a rare adverse disorder called pseudotumor cerebri, or idiopathic intracranial hypertension, (an elevated pressure of the fluid around the brain from an unknown cause) caused by her tetracycline medication[74]. I gave the mother the information I found, obtained the medications for Ashley recommended by the neurologist, and arranged a time for the mother to talk with me in the morning regarding how her daughter was doing.

The following morning the mother related that Ashley did well part of the night but then started to have headaches and double vision again. The mom then brought Ashley to our emergency room for other spinal tap while I arranged for the teenager to be seen by the neurologist as soon as possible. Another spinal tap revealed the initial fluid pressure to be over 500 millimeters again. This time I removed twice as much fluid and the finishing pressure was only 140 millimeters. Ashley felt better instantly, her double vision almost resolved, her headache resolved.

I gave the parents more documentation of my thoughts and an appointment to see the neurologist in a couple days. Since Ashley was an identical twin, it was possible that Allison, or Peanut, would develop the same problem if she received tetracycline antibiotics.

I called Annabelle about Ashley every day until their appointment with the neurologist. In the interim, Ashley started to feel "almost normal" after she had been on the medicines for several days.

The neurologist evaluated both Ashley and Allison. She concluded that the tetracycline medication and not the head trauma from playing basketball was the culprit for Ashley's double vision and headaches. Since it was near the time of the holiday vacation, the neurologist suggested that Ashley not participate in any sports until after the first of the year. She and the parents were strongly advised about ever taking tetracycline antibiotics again for any reason. Subsequently, I contacted the ophthalmologist and the dermatologist regarding Ashley's misadventure.

Except for different medications for their acne and managing various sports injuries, Peanut and Potato flourished. They both graduated with high honors. They both went on to college and excelled in their studies. Becoming dentists, the pair returned to Montana to help others.

Three Monkeys

A fellow medical student and I organized an Oregon summer migrant health program in the summer of 1972. Our job was to arrange for clinic sites, obtain drug samples from pharmaceutical companies, staff the clinics with medical students, and arrange for local physicians to oversee the activities in the clinics. The clinics were placed in the areas of northern Oregon where migrant workers came to harvest various crops. The clinics always operated in the evenings after the workers were done for the day, and for the most part our system worked well with only an occasional glitch. One evening the physician who was supposed to be the preceptor for the clinic did not come. When I called the local hospital to see if he had an emergency, I was told that he was on vacation. He obviously had forgotten to look at his schedule and to notify us so we could find another physician preceptor.

Our clinic was filling up with patients and we, the medical students, had no one to supervise our activities. I made calls to other local physicians to see if I could recruit them on an emergency basis for our clinic. I was not having any luck. On my very last phone call trying to find a local physician to help us, I talked to a doctor's wife at their home. She informed me that her husband was outside nearby cutting trees for an elderly neighbor but she would drive to the neighbor's home and have him return my call. Dr. Ehrlich was a middle-aged general practitioner in the area who I knew enjoyed being with medical students. Perhaps ten minutes later Dr. Ehrlich was on the phone wanting to know what he could do to help, and I informed him of our dilemma. In turn, he told me of his dilemma, which was that he had promised his neighbor for weeks that he would cut down her old trees. He told me he was dirty as hell and definitely not presentable to be in a clinic seeing patients. He then paused a few moments and finally said in frustration, "Oh hell, I'll tell my neighbor the trees will have to wait for another day. People are more important than dead trees." Dr. Ehrlich then said he could be at the clinic in fifteen minutes, so we could go ahead and start seeing patients. He thought we could catch up in short order. The rest of the evening in the clinic was uneventful. In appreciation for his generosity, the staff at the clinic and the medical students all pitched in a few dollars each for Dr. Ehrlich to take his wife to dinner.

In the late afternoon on a Saturday in late summer of 1978 I was working in my garden when Kay summoned me to the phone. She said it was the emergency room nurse wanting to talk to me. Walking across the yard to the house, I told Kay that I was not on call. Elizabeth, the nurse on duty in the emergency room that Saturday, told me that the doctor on call could not be found and none of the other doctors in town were willing to come to the emergency room. She was hoping that I would come or else she was going to have to transfer her patients to fifty miles away Williston, North Dakota, for treatment. I recalled Dr. Ehrlich's comments in 1972 that people were more important than trees. In my case, I thought people were more important than weeding my garden. Besides, we were trying to improve the image of our hospital, and sending trauma patients away to a nearby hospital would indeed be bad public relations in a small community.

Elizabeth told me that there were three young boys in the emergency room who had been injured trying to ride a cow. She told me I could take my time driving the five miles from my home into town because all the boys were stable and Jack, the x-ray technician, was taking pictures of anything that was bent or hurt. Elizabeth had been a nurse for a long time and I trusted her judgment implicitly. When I arrived in the emergency room Elizabeth directed me to the x-ray department where the three patients were still being processed. Subsequently, I walked the short distance to radiology where I could examine them.

The three boys were cousins between nine and twelve years old. All had tears running down their faces, but not one of them was making a sound. As I was about to examine the first boy, a

woman walked into the x-ray department and identified herself
as one of the boys' mothers. She told me that the three little cowboys had decided to ride a cow. Not an old lazy almost ready to
die cow, but a five-month-old full-of-energy calf. Apparently, the
boys managed to get the calf into a cattle chute with one end
open. The three then mounted the calf and held on for dear life.
The mother did not see the incident and admitted that she was
just relaying the story that she pieced together from the little
boys. The youngster that was least injured ran up to the house
on the ranch and brought the mother down to the corrals. She
found two of the boys lying on the ground moaning. The mother
noticed that the calf appeared to be uninjured. The woman said
she then loaded up the three into the pickup truck and drove the
twenty-five miles into town.

On examination, one boy had been knocked out and had an
obvious concussion. He had a linear bruise across his forehead
where he apparently hit one of the rails of the cattle chute. A second boy had a slight deformity of his left forearm, which x-rays
revealed to be a small fracture near the wrist. I knew this type of
fracture in a child this age would require just a cast for a couple
weeks. The third boy had multiple superficial abrasions on his
arms and shoulders. He did not know what happened to him, but
I surmised that he was thrown into the air and landed on his
back in the dirt.

After I reassured the mother that all three boys were going to
be okay, she started to sing a modified version of the bedtime
tune *Five Little Monkeys*:

Three little monkeys jumping on a cow,
One fell off and broke his crown.
Mama called the Doctor and the Doctor said,
"That's what you get for jumping on a cow!"

Before coming to town, the woman sent one of her ranch
hands to notify the boys' fathers who were brothers and were

working mending fences somewhere on the ranch. About the time the boys were ready to be discharged from the emergency room, the two fathers arrived. Coming down the hallway in the hospital they heard the song about three monkeys. Entering the emergency room one of the men said, "So these are the three monkeys who tried to ride a calf." The two men walked around looking at the boys' injuries, and deciding that they were not too bad, asked if the calf was hurt. Before the boys could reply, the brothers looked at each other and one said, "Seems to me there's a lot of corrals on the ranch that need to be painted by three little monkeys with not much to do and who want to be cowboys." The other cowboy agreed. The two men then turned around and as they were walking out the emergency room door told the woman there was work to be done and they would be home for supper. The painting would start first thing in the morning.

The three little monkeys did not say a word.

White as Snow

On a wintry day in 1978, Elizabeth Hanratty brought her three-year-old son Henry into my office for me to evaluate the pain in his ears. Henry spent his days in the day care center where, according to the mother, the kids had been sick all winter. Just like the other kids in the day care center Henry's nose had been congested for weeks and was constantly draining discolored mucous. Finally, the night before our visit, Henry complained of pain in both ears and cried most of the evening. In the morning before coming to the office Elizabeth noticed that gray green goo started to come out of Henry's left ear and he appeared to be more comfortable.

My evaluation of Henry revealed a little boy with a mild upper respiratory infection with associated infections in both ears. The left eardrum had opened from the pressure of the infection behind it (called an internal otitis) and a thick discolored material was draining onto the outside portion of the ear. This area was inflamed and infected also (called an external otitis). I knew that a short course of oral antibiotics and some local care to the outside ear should clear up both ear infections. The remainder of his upper respiratory illness was caused by a virus and would resolve soon.

Elizabeth also brought her five-year-old daughter Heather along this day because she could not find a babysitter on such a short notice. I observed that Heather seemed pale when I contrasted her skin to her very dark brown hair. I asked the mother if she would mind if I looked at Heather while she was there. Somewhat puzzled, Elizabeth told me that Heather was not the sick child, but she allowed me to examine the youngster anyhow.

As Heather sat quietly on a chair in the examination room I saw that she appeared tired and moved slowly when I asked her to get up on the examination table. Again, I was struck by the paleness of Heather's skin and asked her mother if this color of her skin was unusual. Elizabeth had not noticed anything unusual.

The color under the fingernails should be pink in a healthy individual. Usually, when the tip of a fingernail is depressed, the pink tissue under the nail blanches. When the pressure is released, the pink coloration returns briskly. I initially noticed that Heather's fingernails were also pale. When I pressed on the tip of the fingernail, the tissue underneath did not blanch, and I knew instantly this child was substantially anemic for some reason. I thought only of the worst diagnoses including leukemia because that is what we doctors do. Further examination revealed only a resting rapid heart rate and a mild heart murmur.

I told Mrs. Hanratty that I thought that her little girl was quite anemic, and I asked for her permission to do a simple blood test to confirm my suspicions. Even though she was puzzled by my comments, the mother allowed me to do the blood test on Heather.

I had our lab technician perform a test called a CBC, or complete blood count, which provides quick and simple information about the number and quality of the cells in a person's blood. In Heather's case, the test revealed a hemoglobin of only four grams when I would have expected twelve grams or more in a child this age. This proved to me that this little girl had a potentially serious anemia for an unknown reason. Additionally, according to the lab's pathologist, all the other components of Heather's blood count appeared normal under the microscope.

I advised Elizabeth of my findings and told her that I was going to consult a pediatric specialist in blood diseases in Seattle before she left my office. Appearing more concerned now that her child might be seriously ill, Elizabeth was more than willing to wait a little longer while I talked with a specialist.

I discussed the case with a pediatric hematology specialist at the University of Washington Medical School who asked me a series of questions regarding Heather's state of health and whether or not I noticed any congenital abnormalities. After I presented Heather's case including the laboratory data, the doctor asked what I thought my patient's problem was. I told him that Heather could have an early leukemia or a disorder called TEC, or transient erythrocytopenia of childhood[72,73]. I had never seen a case of TEC, but I had learned in medical school just a few years before that the disease was first reported in the medical literature around 1970 just as I was entering medical school.

The cells in the bone marrow that produce red blood cells are called erythroblasts. Occasionally, these bone marrow cells dramatically slow down or halt the production of red blood cells, called erythrocytes, with the result being a severe anemia. This curiosity occurs in about one in 200,000 children, and experts believe it to be related to some sort of viral infection. Originally this disorder was termed pure red cell aplasia of children, or PRCAC, when it was thought to be associated with more serious blood disorders like leukemia. After it was determined that the bone marrow cells eventually started producing red blood cells normally again, the disorder was renamed transient erythrocytopenia of childhood or TEC. (Don't we doctors get to play with wonderful terms?) Over time after more cases had been encountered and reported, it appears that the disorder is self-limited and usually resolves within several months, but occasionally it will take up to eighteen months for the child's blood counts to return to the normal values.

The hematologist told me that my diagnosis of TEC could be a very real possibility. Since the child was not acutely ill, the doctor recommended that I give my patient a blood transfusion to increase her blood count about nine grams and then wait. He noted that if my diagnosis was correct, the youngster would be cured within a month or two, otherwise her blood counts would begin to go down again. If the transfusion worked, no more treatment would ever be needed. The doctor asked me to give the mother his name and phone number for consultation if she wished.

I returned to the examination room and discussed my conversation with Elizabeth. I also gave her the name and phone number of the pediatric blood specialist I had consulted at the University of Washington Medical School. Afterward, with the mother's permission, Heather received a blood transfusion at the hospital.

I checked Heather's blood count every two weeks for the next few months and sent the information to the pediatrician at the University of Washington Medical School. Not only did Heather's blood count not decrease, but it increased over time, thus confirming the diagnosis. According to the mother, Heather's energy level increased substantially.

I had the opportunity to watch Heather for another twenty years. The anemia did not return.

Temporary Blindness

After I retired from medical practice I decided to learn how to play golf. Before long others persuaded me to play in a senior men's golf league. When I told the league organizers that I was finished with highly competitive sports, they assured me that the senior men's league was anything but highly competitive. They told me the golf league consisted of just a bunch of old men looking for fellowship and having a good time at the golf course. The ages of the men ranged from about sixty to ninety-two.

I signed up for the Monday morning senior men's league. Maynard, one of the league organizers, handed me a scorecard for my first round of golf to be played with other seniors. He told me I got to keep score for our foursome and then with a big grin on his face Maynard said, "When you're done I want you to tell me how competitive your round was. Have a good time."

I thought Maynard had made it easy on me by having my foursome start on the very first hole, but I soon realized as we were becoming acquainted before the match that I had three interesting companions. The first golfer was deaf even with hearing aids in both ears. The second golfer had severe dementia with a short-term recall of nanoseconds and would be riding in the golf cart driven by the deaf first golfer. The third golfer had severe macular degeneration, was essentially blind, and would be my partner. You can imagine the four of us trying to communicate as we played a round of golf. The deaf man relied upon the man with dementia to give him instructions. Since the man with dementia couldn't remember anything, his instructions were usually wrong. Meanwhile, the man with dementia thought all the golf balls on the golf course belonged to him, and he would take off by himself in the golf cart picking up other players' golf balls. My partner could barely see his ball on the ground and frequently missed it by inches in all directions as he took his swings.

Obviously, my group spent a lot of time trying to find lost golf balls, and certainly we did not win the tournament.

When we finished the round of golf, I met Maynard in the clubhouse who asked me laughing with a big cheesy smile on his face how competitive the golf round was. I knew I was the object of his big joke for the day. I told Maynard that I had a very interesting day and that unfortunately, despite our very best efforts, we took last place by a large margin. Maynard smiled and said, "Doc, see you next week." I chuckled to myself as I thought about all the maladies of aging that may be awaiting me.

Soon after I started playing in the league and other players became aware that I was a physician in my working days, I became Doc. Since most of the players were old enough not to recall names very well, Doc was easy to remember. While playing with senior citizen men I soon realized that there was still a need for my services and opinions. The players often have questions about surgical operations, medicines, general information about disease processes, and what I thought in general about where medicine was today. I took it all in stride since it made me feel still useful.

The summer sky was bright and cloudless with a gorgeous clear Montana Big Sky Monday morning in July at 8 o'clock when we started off on the tenth tee box. One of the players in our foursome was eighty-year-old Godfrey Morton. As we were becoming acquainted that morning, one of the other golfers took me aside and informed me that Godfrey was a hypochondriac. The golfer told me that every time he played with Godfrey the man managed to have a new illness, or a new pill, or wondered if he should have another operation to relieve a mysterious illness. The golfer just wanted me to know that I had been forewarned and not get too carried away when talking with Godfrey.

When I introduced myself to Godfrey he told me that he understood I was a doctor. When I told him that I had been a family physician in a rural area and had seen and done many things in medicine, Godfrey started to talk about one of his ailments. The other two golfers implored Godfrey to just hit the ball. Unfortunately, one of the other golfers recognized that Godfrey was now using yellow golf balls instead of white ones. Before teeing off, Godfrey explained to us that his eye doctor told him he was going blind from macular degeneration and he might see the yellow balls better. Just that morning Godfrey purchased a box of a dozen brand-new Titleist yellow golf balls for about fifty dollars. He made sure all of us knew he was playing expensive golf balls that morning.

The weather was wonderful and the pace of play was good this particular morning. As luck would have it, the sky became overcast and dark ominous clouds started to arrive after about an hour. A storm was brewing, a brisk wind started to blow, and it became increasingly dark by the time we reached the tee box for the par 3 seventeenth hole. When Godfrey got up for his turn to hit, he placed a bright yellow ball on a tee, took out his club, and addressed the ball. He waited standing beside his ball getting positioned for what seemed a long time. The other golfers reminded Godfrey that time was wasting and to hit the ball.

Godfrey stepped back and told us that he was having difficulty focusing on the ball. He asked us to be patient for just a moment. Then Godfrey reached into his golf bag and pulled out his new pair of blue-blocker sunglasses with yellow lenses. He informed us that his eye doctor told him that with his macular degeneration he would be able to see better on dark days if he used this type of sunglasses. Godfrey bragged that he just paid one hundred fifty dollars for these fancy prescription sunglasses. Thinking he was just having another one of his hypochondriacal episodes, one of the other golfers pleaded with Gottfried to just HIT THE BALL!

Godfrey's ball was still mounted on a tee as he donned his new yellow colored sunglasses and stood to address the golf ball. We were expecting something miraculous, but Godfrey did not move. While the other golfers were coaxing Godfrey to hit the ball, he

stood motionless with his face pointed at the ground and did not
say a word in retaliation to the coaxing. Godfrey then took a step
back, leaned on his golf club, and exclaimed, "I'm having a stroke!
I'm blind. I can't see a damn thing! I can't see the ball!"

One of the other golfers was incredulous and exclaimed, "Oh
for crying out loud. Here we go again!"

I knew, however, that Godfrey could not go blind in both eyes
in an instant without having some other symptoms and tried to
reassure him.

One of the other golfers was holding his white golf ball and
dropped it next to Godfrey's ball. He asked Godfrey if he could
see his white golf ball. When Godfrey replied that he could, the
other golfers said in unison, "Well hit the damn thing."

Now Godfrey was in a dilemma. He could see the white golf
ball but he couldn't see his expensive yellow golf ball. He stood on
the tee box mumbling to himself, "What is going on?"

I asked Godfrey to take off his glasses and instantly he saw
both golf balls. Godfrey asserted, "I'm only blind some of the time
I guess."

I suggested that he was trying to see a yellow ball through
yellow tinted glasses. That was the only problem. He did not
have a stroke. One of the other golfers gave Godfrey a brand-new
white golf ball to hit while wearing his expensive yellow sunglasses with the admonition to just, "Hit the damn ball before we
get caught in a storm."

Godfrey replaced his yellow ball with the white ball, carefully
donned his yellow sunglasses so he could see better, and then
promptly hit the brand new golf ball into the lake. What more
could we say?

Godfrey finished playing the last two holes with borrowed
used white golf balls while wearing his expensive yellow blue-
blocker sunglasses. Our foursome finished playing just before
lightning, thunder, rain, severe winds and hail closed the golf
course. In the clubhouse eighty-year-old Godfrey continued to
ruminate aloud about whether he should play with his expensive

yellow golf balls or his expensive yellow sunglasses. Needing to relieve some stress, the other golfers headed to the bar for a beer. I had my usual, a Dr. Pepper of course.

In the early afternoon sometime in late August I was about to start a round of golf when I felt a tap on my right shoulder. Instinctively, I turned and before I knew it someone had grabbed my hand and was shaking it. Then I heard, "Hey Doc, remember me?" Before I could say a word the man continued, "You have to remember me. I'm Godfrey Morton, the guy who thought he was having a stroke when he couldn't see his yellow golf ball."

I answered that I recalled that day very well, and I was glad he did not have a stroke.

Mr. Morton then went on to tell me that he went back to see his eye doctor who told him that he also was colorblind. Godfrey explained that his eye doctor informed him that, "His mother gave him colorblindness when he was a child." Consequently, the yellow glasses with the yellow ball in a colorblind person meant he could not see the golf ball.

I tried to be cordial and nodded my head in appreciation of his comments without saying a word. I did not have the heart to tell Godfrey that his mother did not give him colorblindness but rather he was born with it, and he had been colorblind his entire life. About fifteen percent of all men have colorblindness, a genetic trait from which only one of the genes comes from the mother and none from the father.

Godfrey said he was in a hurry, but as he was walking away he just wanted to thank me for caring about him that day before the storm. He told me that now on sunny days he uses yellow balls, and on cloudy days he uses his yellow sunglasses with white balls. As he was getting into his golf cart, Godfrey proclaimed that he knew his golf game was going to improve now that he had a brand-new set of golf clubs that cost him twelve hundred dollars.

I knew it wasn't so, but I applauded him for his optimism at age eighty.

Hey Doc, Remember Me?

Around the time of my retirement from medical practice I was browsing in a department store in Billings, Montana, when I thought I heard my name called. It was a busy weekend day in the department store and when I looked around to see who was calling all I could see were the heads of many people. Therefore, I continued browsing.

Before long I heard, "Doc Ashcraft, Doc Ashcraft, it's me!"

Again, I scanned the store 360° to see who was calling my name. Still I saw nobody familiar. I continued shopping.

Once more a man's voice called out, "Doctor Ashcraft! Doctor Ashcraft! Hey Doc, remember me?"

This time when I looked around the store I saw a pair of arms waving madly above the crowd perhaps one hundred feet away. I soon noticed that the arms were connected to a tall middle-aged man with bushy red hair who was literally running down the aisle calling my name. The man stopped running as he approached me and being somewhat winded shouted, "Hey Doc, remember me? I'm Jeremy Patterson. Do you remember me now?" He extended his hand for a handshake.

As I was shaking the man's hand, I had to confess to him that I did not have a clue who he was. I asked him to refresh my memory.

Turning his head to the right to display his left ear, the man grabbed his ear with his left hand and wiggled it. He then said, "Do you remember me now?"

I told the man that neither his face nor his ear rang a bell in my memory banks. I could only apologize for my lack of recall.

The man quickly told me that during the winter of 1977 during the oil boom he was only nineteen years old and was working on a drilling rig near Alexander, North Dakota. One weekend when they were not working, he and some friends battled the snowdrifts and the cold weather to drive thirty miles into Sidney, Montana, to have some fun. Mr. Patterson admitted that he and his friends went barhopping in Sidney, and when they got to the Mint Bar and Cafe sometime after midnight they were pretty drunk. It was not unusual for underage oil workers to receive alcohol during the oil boom. As long as the men had a pocket full of money, few checked to see how old they were. At the Mint Bar one thing led to another as things do when men unaccustomed to alcohol drink too much. Before he knew it, Jeremy and his friends were fighting with some other oilfield workers. Loud talk turned into a pushing match, which turned into fisticuffs that ended in someone pulling a knife on Mr. Patterson and nearly cutting off his left ear. The man told me that his compatriots dragged him to the hospital emergency room and later told him that his ear was hanging by a thread. He told me that I was the one who sewed his ear back on in the wee hours of that morning at the local hospital.

I asked him if I could check out the results of my handiwork after almost thirty years.

Mr. Patterson said it would be his pleasure to show me his battle scars. He took his right arm and pulled his left ear forward so I could see the very fine scar between the backside of his ear and his skull. The man wiggled his ear back and forth with his hand to show me that it was firmly attached. He then said, "Doc, looks like you did a pretty good job!" Mr. Patterson then commented that his fiancée at the time would not have married him if he were missing a left ear. He then smiled and chuckled to himself.

I told Mr. Patterson that I still did not recall the incident since it was so long ago and I saw so many trauma patients in the emergency room during those years, but I was glad that he had a good result.

Mr. Patterson then told me that it may have been just another day at the office for me but it meant an awful lot to him. He thanked me for doing such a good job on a drunk so many years before.

I acknowledged his thoughtful comments, shook his hand, and away he went back into the crowd. It has always amazed me how such apparently insignificant incidents for me, or other doctors, made lasting memories for our patients.

Final Thoughts

For someone well past the midpoint of his seventh decade, I have found that hitting a little white ball on a golf course can be almost as emotionally satisfying as delivering a healthy newborn baby or rescuing someone from the brink of death in the emergency room. I enjoy playing golf alone because it allows me plenty of time to think as I walk down the fairways. Recently, as I was considering writing this book, I thought about many of the things that I experienced in medicine during my lifetime and wanted to share some of my thoughts, memories, experiences, and recollections from the last half-century or so.

As a child in the late 1950s I recall receiving an injection of penicillin in my butt from Dr. P. E. Wally when I had a severe case of tonsillitis, and my fever and my throat pain were a lot better the next day when Dr. Wally returned to my home to check on me. He advised my parents to have my tonsils removed, but they declined, and I still have my tonsils today. With what I know now about bacterial throat infections, I wonder about whether or not I would have developed rheumatic fever with its associated heart valve damage had I not received the injection of penicillin. For Dr. Wally, who was not a young man as I recall, the introduction of penicillin into his medical practice must have been a godsend.

Inexplicably, when I was starting the seventh grade, I decided I wanted to be a doctor. Here I was, a little runt of a kid telling people I wanted to become a doctor. My parents never had any leftover money, and certainly they would never have any money to help me go to college, much less medical school. My parents and essentially all of my many relatives never completed high school nor did many of my classmates. But I wanted to be a doctor, and with luck and a lot of help along the way, I made it.

As a freshman medical student in 1970, I spent many evenings learning about and caring for sick babies in the newborn intensive care unit at the Doernbecher Children's Hospital on the campus of the University of Oregon Medical School in Portland, Oregon. Doctors from all over the region sent their premature babies to the medical school in hopes that the best pediatricians in the area could save the infants struggling to breathe with respiratory distress, which was termed hyaline membrane disease at the time. Despite the best efforts of the doctors and the nurses, most of the premature infants died because doctors just did not know the cause of, or how to treat, diseases of the immature lungs of the premature baby. In the late 1980s, a biologic preparation called surfactant was discovered and became available to treat the lung disease of the premature infant by enabling normal physiology in the lungs. Instead of losing ten thousand to fifteen thousand babies a year from premature lung disease, only one in a thousand sick babies would die from premature lung disease by 2010. Surfactant[75] was indeed an amazing discovery for pediatrics.

In 1970, the chance of dying from anesthesia given during a surgical operation could be as high as three thousand deaths per one hundred thousand cases or three percent. With new anesthesia agents and improved protocols, the chance of such deaths in 2015 when I had surgery was only about 0.5 deaths in one hundred thousand cases.

The developments in heart surgery in the 1960s and 70s to replace valves damaged by rheumatic fever and aging improved the lives and increased the lifespans of many. Unfortunately, the enthusiasm for heart bypass surgery several decades later never underwent controlled clinical evaluations, and after about twenty-five years of this surgery, the long-term morbidity and mortality data revealed that many people lived just as long by just taking some medication. Cardiologists gradually developed safer and less expensive procedures to implant small tubes called stents into the diseased arteries of the heart that supplanted the majority of heart bypass surgery. We should know the long-term results from these newer less-invasive procedures in another generation. However, the initial outcome data are favorable.

The invention and development of the microcomputer since the late 1970s revolutionized all endeavors in our lives including healthcare. Electronic gizmos of all sorts are now available to diagnose, treat, and help patients in essentially all specialties of medicine. Developing computers' capability to process immense amount of data unraveled life's genetic code and now can be used to determine individual patients' genetic codes in a matter of hours instead of years. The microcomputer enables physicians to access promptly the worldwide medical literature at the bedside. My note taking in medical school with a pen and paper has been supplanted by lectures presented on laptop computer screens sent from another electronic source. Unfortunately, in my opinion, the computer at the bedside is just another hindrance to the very personal doctor-patient relationship. Today's doctors seem to be more interested in generating data for a computer databank than paying attention to their patients. With my experiences as a medical student, a patient, a practicing physician, and a medical faculty educator, I know that my training in clinical medicine was much better than the experience medical students receive today.

Doctors have learned the hard way that all that is written in respected medical journals cannot be trusted. Our profession depends upon honest, accurate, up-to-date research information. When a single fraudulent case study was reported in the *New England Journal of Medicine* in the 1980s, most scientists and physicians wrote it off as a single bad apple in the honorable profession of scientific research. However, as the years passed, additional important studies proved to be flawed or outright fraud. When the long time editors of two of the world's most prestigious medical journals, the *New England Journal of Medicine* and the *Lancet*, spoke out about the poor quality of clinical research, many were astounded.[76] Physicians now must be more careful than ever when differentiating between the information they receive as important, relevant, or downright bogus before they use it to care for patients.

I guess many in my profession did not have the luxury to be taught science by teachers like Fred Kayser who noted, "Science was about being accurate and being truthful, not about being wishful."

With so many places to obtain medical information on the worldwide web that may be good, bad, harmful, or indifferent, patients still must rely on their physicians to provide them with accurate health information and honest advice. In my view, the internet, even though it has many good attributes, has become yet another obstacle interfering with the personal relationship between a doctor and a patient.

Any person of science knows that there must be balance. For every positive there must be a negative. For every right there must be a left. For every up there must be a down. For every good there must be a bad. In the past half-century those in healthcare have done a lot of good; they have also done a lot of bad. Infant mortality is now approaching zero when it was near twenty percent in 1900[77]. Many in medicine would like to take credit for this achievement. Unfortunately, the credit really belongs to increasing our understanding about germs, to the development of adequate sanitation systems, to the increased use of soap and water, and to the reliable availability of clean water supplies. On the other end of the spectrum, in rich nations and in poor nations, people around the world are living much longer, filling up nursing homes, and costing societies mightily. Humans are the only biologic population on earth to spend more resources on the elderly than on the young.

Over the past half century I have seen and experienced many changes in medicine. Whether the changes are considered good or bad will require much more time, but here are some of my personal observations:

1. Medical care has become de-personalized. The calling that I had and still feel for medicine has become just another job for many.

2. Having health insurance and a computerized medical record will not make one healthy.

3. Patients have an insatiable desire for healthcare services as long as someone else pays the bills.

4. The interventions of government policy, insurance payers, the media, and the legal system have produced unrealistic expectations from patients regarding their illnesses.

5. Maintaining one's health and managing complex illnesses are difficult problems. Solutions are never simple or easy despite what patients and doctors desire.

6. Patients and many doctors believe that no one should ever be sick or have pain. For many in America death is considered an option. It is not.

7. A compassionate death with dignity at home surrounded by loved ones a few days earlier is far better than a mechanized, agonizing death alone in an intensive care unit.

Today's doctors learn differently than I did back in the day. A single computer tablet has replaced all the pencils, paper, chalkboards, and slide rules of my era. A computer connected to the internet has replaced the innumerable hours I spent looking up, finding, and reading books and magazines in the library. My young grandchildren do not spend time in school learning to write with a pen or pencil because in the future everything will be on computers and a person's identification signature will be either a fingerprint, an eyeball scan, or something else. A finger touch to the bottom of a computer screen flipping book pages has replaced the wonderful tactile stimulation I get by turning a book's paper pages. This is the future of education today. Is it better? Only time will tell. I do know that the medical students and doctors of today need to learn a lot more "stuff" than I did.

However, a more important question might be, "Are they learning enough of the right stuff to be good doctors that can provide compassionate care to their patients?"

Some children have never been to a library to locate and enjoy a real book. Many think they're going to a museum, and perhaps they are. Now I am one of the nostalgic dinosaurs in the museum sitting in a chair reading one of those thick paper things.

Many people, patients and physicians alike, have come to believe, and indeed expect, that the human body can be made to last a century before it finally collapses suddenly into a pile of dust much like the wonderful one-hoss shay in Oliver Wendall Holmes' 1858 classic poem *The Deacon's Masterpiece*.[78,79] This longevity and instant demise supposedly occurs without the human body experiencing any disease, any decreases in function, without having pain, and without any suffering. These ideas are obviously fantasy. As I have experienced in my later years, the natural aging process sadly does not unfold so simply. (For those of you who have wondered about the logical poem *The Deacon's Masterpiece or The Wonderful One-Hoss Shay*, but have never read it, I have included a copy of it at the end of the book for your enjoyment.)

Well, the sun is out, the Montana Big Sky is clear, the wind is mild, the temperature is just right, and the fairways at the nearby golf course are beckoning me. I think its time for another leisurely stroll down a groomed grassy road with a metal stick and a small white ball to do more thinking about the balance in nature. There is a lake beside the 15th fairway tempting my golf ball to join it for a swim, again.

The Deacon's Masterpiece (1858)
by Oliver Wendell Holmes, Sr.

Have you heard of the wonderful one-hoss shay,
That was built in such a logical way
It ran a hundred years to a day,
And then, of a sudden, it — ah, but stay,
I'll tell you what happened without delay,
Scaring the parson into fits,
Frightening people out of their wits, —
Have you ever heard of that, I say?

Seventeen hundred and fifty-five.
Georgius Secundus was then alive, —
Snuffy old drone from the German hive.
That was the year when Lisbon-town
Saw the earth open and gulp her down,
And Braddock's army was done so brown,
Left without a scalp to its crown.
It was on the terrible Earthquake-day
That the Deacon finished the one-hoss shay.

Now in building of chaises, I tell you what,
There is always *somewhere* a weakest spot, —
In hub, tire, felloe, in spring or thill,
In panel, or crossbar, or floor, or sill,
In screw, bolt, thoroughbrace, — lurking still,
Find it somewhere you must and will, —
Above or below, or within or without, —
And that's the reason, beyond a doubt,
A chaise *breaks down*, but doesn't *wear out*.

But the Deacon swore (as Deacons do,
With an "I dew vum," or an "I tell yeou")
He would build one shay to beat the taown

'N' the keounty 'n' all the kentry raoun';
It should be so built that it *could n'* break daown:
"Fur," said the Deacon, "'t 's mighty plain
Thut the weakes' place mus' stan' the strain;
'N' the way t' fix it, uz I maintain,
    Is only jest
T' make that place uz strong uz the rest."

So the Deacon inquired of the village folk
Where he could find the strongest oak,
That could n't be split nor bent nor broke, —
That was for spokes and floor and sills;
He sent for lancewood to make the thills;
The crossbars were ash, from the straightest trees,
The panels of white-wood, that cuts like cheese,
But lasts like iron for things like these;
The hubs of logs from the "Settler's ellum," —
Last of its timber, — they could n't sell 'em,
Never an axe had seen their chips,
And the wedges flew from between their lips,
Their blunt ends frizzled like celery-tips;
Step and prop-iron, bolt and screw,
Spring, tire, axle, and linchpin too,
Steel of the finest, bright and blue;
Thoroughbrace bison-skin, thick and wide;
Boot, top, dasher, from tough old hide
Found in the pit when the tanner died.
That was the way he "put her through."
"There!" said the Deacon, "naow she'll dew!"

Do! I tell you, I rather guess
She was a wonder, and nothing less!
Colts grew horses, beards turned gray,
Deacon and deaconess dropped away,
Children and grandchildren — where were they?

But there stood the stout old one-hoss shay
As fresh as on Lisbon-earthquake-day!

EIGHTEEN HUNDRED; — it came and found
The Deacon's masterpiece strong and sound.
Eighteen hundred increased by ten; —
"Hahnsum kerridge" they called it then.
Eighteen hundred and twenty came; —
Running as usual; much the same.
Thirty and forty at last arrive,
And then come fifty, and FIFTY-FIVE.

Little of all we value here
Wakes on the morn of its hundreth year
Without both feeling and looking queer.
In fact, there's nothing that keeps its youth,
So far as I know, but a tree and truth.
(This is a moral that runs at large;
Take it. — You're welcome. — No extra charge.)

FIRST OF NOVEMBER, — the Earthquake-day, —
There are traces of age in the one-hoss shay,
A general flavor of mild decay,
But nothing local, as one may say.
There could n't be, — for the Deacon's art
Had made it so like in every part
That there was n't a chance for one to start.
For the wheels were just as strong as the thills,
And the floor was just as strong as the sills,
And the panels just as strong as the floor,
And the whipple-tree neither less nor more,
And the back crossbar as strong as the fore,
And spring and axle and hub *encore*.
And yet, *as a whole*, it is past a doubt
In another hour it will be *worn out*!

First of November, 'Fifty-five!
This morning the parson takes a drive.
Now, small boys, get out of the way!
Here comes the wonderful one-hoss shay,
Drawn by a rat-tailed, ewe-necked bay.
"Huddup!" said the parson. — Off went they.
The parson was working his Sunday's text, —
Had got to *fifthly*, and stopped perplexed
At what the — Moses — was coming next.
All at once the horse stood still,
Close by the meet'n'-house on the hill.
First a shiver, and then a thrill,
Then something decidedly like a spill, —
And the parson was sitting upon a rock,
At half past nine by the meet'n-house clock, —
Just the hour of the Earthquake shock!
What do you think the parson found,
When he got up and stared around?
The poor old chaise in a heap or mound,
As if it had been to the mill and ground!
You see, of course, if you're not a dunce,
How it went to pieces all at once, —
All at once, and nothing first, —
Just as bubbles do when they burst.

End of the wonderful one-hoss shay.
Logic is logic. That's all I say.

Bibliography

General References:

Blaser, Martin, MD, *Missing Microbes*, Picador, 2014

Brill, Steven, *America's Bitter Pill*, Random House, 2015

Clapesattle, Helen, *The Doctors Mayo*, Mayo Foundation, 1969

DeGowin & DeGowin, *Bedside Diagnostic Evaluation*, Macmillan, 1969

Harrison's Principles of Internal Medicine, Sixth edition, McGraw-Hill, 1970

Harrison's Principles of Internal Medicine, Seventeenth edition, McGraw-Hill, 2008

National Center for Health Statistics, http://www.cdc.gov/nchs/

National Library of Medicine, http://www.ncbi.nlm.nih.gov

National Vital Statistics Reports, http://www.cdc.gov/nchs/products/nvsr.htm

Reilly, Brendan, MD, *One Doctor*, Simon and Schuster, 2013

Wikipedia, the internet encyclopedia, http://www.wikipedia.org/

Introduction:
1. What Happened in 1960, http://www.thepeoplehistory.com/1960.html

2. Yellowstone Wolves Changed The Entire Ecosystem, Even The Geography, Inquisitr, May 17,2015, http://www.inquisitr.com/2091814/

3. How Wolves Change Rivers - YouTube,
   www.youtube.com/watch?v=ysa5OBhXz-Q

4. Quake Lake, Wikipedia

5. Martin Blaser, MD, *Missing Microbes*, Picador, 2014

A Bump in the Road:
6. Methicillin, Wikipedia

7. MRSA, www.cdc.gov/mrsa/

8. The Hospitalist, Hospital Medicine,
   https://en.wikipedia.org/wiki/Hospital_medicine

9. Mycosis Fungoides, *Harrison's Principles of Internal Medicine*, 1970

10. Mycosis Fungoides, *Harrison's Principles of Internal Medicine*, 2008

Emergency Department:
11. Tang et al, Trends and Characteristics of US Emergency Department Visits, 1997-2007; JAMA, 2010 August 11, 304(6); 664-670, http://www.ncbi.nlm.nih.gov

12. FastStats - Emergency Department Visits, AHRQ, www.cdc.gov Trends in Emergency Department Visits, 2006-2011, Skinner, et al

13. ER Visits Continue to Rise Since Implementation of the Affordable Care Act, ACEP, May 4, 2015, newsroom.acep.org/2015-05...

The Kids' Surgeon:
14. Knope, Steven, MD, Libby Zion: The Day Medicine changed Forever, Nov. 7, https://en.wikipedia.org/wiki/Libby_Zion_Law 2013, www.conciergemedicinemd.com/blog/2013/11/07

15. From the Death of Libby Zion, Crucial Medical Reforms, www.nytimes.com/2009/03/03/health/03zion.html

Martha:
16. Christakis and Lamont, Extent and determinants of error in doctors' prognoses in terminally ill patients: prospective cohort study; British Medical Journal, 2000 Feb 19;320(7233):469-72, http://www.ncbi.nlm.nih.gov/pubmed/10678857

17. Lamont and Christakis, Prognostic Disclosure to Patients with Cancer Near the End of Life, Annals of Internal Medicine 2001;134:1096.

18. Ubel, Peter, Truth in the Most Optimistic Way, Annals of Internal Medicine 2001;134:142; annals.org/article.aspx?articleid=714572

19. The high Cost of Cancer Care, Your Money or Your Life, www.newsweek.com

20. Beil, Laura, The Cancer "Breakthroughs" that Cost Too Much and Do Too Little, Newsweek, August 27, 2012 , The Cancer "Breakthroughs" that Cost Too Much and Do Too Little

21. Smith,R, Editor In Chief Of World's Best Known Medical Journal: Half …,May 16, 2015, www.collective-evolution.com/.../editor-in-chief-of-worlds-best-known-Peer review: a flawed process at the heart of science and journals,2006,www.ncbi.nlm.nih.gov/.

22. The Ethical Nag, Marcia Angell, http://ethicalnag.org/2009/11/09/nejm-editor/

Lars:
23. Home Care, Wikipedia, https://en.wikipedia.org/wiki/Home_care

24. History of Home Care, http://www.pinnaclehomecare.net/homecarehis.html

25. History of Hospice Care, http://www.nhpco.org/history-hospice-care

26. What is the history of hospice?
    https://en.wikipedia.org/wiki/Home_care

I Can't Walk:
27. Guillain-Barré, Wikipedia

28. Guillain-Barré, *Harrison's Principles of Internal Medicine*,
    Sixth edition, McGraw- Hill, 1970

29. Guillain-Barré, *Harrison's Principles of Internal Medicine*,
    Seventeenth edition, McGraw-Hill, 2008

30. Guillain-Barré Syndrome Fact Sheet,
    http://www.ninds.nih.gov/disorders/gbs/detailgbs.htm

A Hometown Hero:
31. Statistics and Outlook for cancer of the larynx,
    http://www.cancerresearchuk.org/about-cancer/type/larynx-
    cancer/treatment/statistics-and-outlook-for-cancer-of-the-
    larynx

32. Head and neck cancer, Wikipedia,
    https://en.wikipedia.org/wiki/Head_and_neck_cancer

The Catheter:
33. Pollock, Richard, Doctors, hospitals rethinking electronic
    medical records, Washington Examiner, October 10, 2014,
    http://www.washingtonexaminer.com/doctors-hospitals-
    rethinking-electronic-medical-records- mandated-by-2009-
    law/article/2554622

The Biker:
34. Infective endocarditis,
    https://en.wikipedia.org/wiki/Infective_endocarditis

35. Bacterial endocarditis, *Bedside Diagnostic Evaluation*,
    DeGowin & DeGowin, Macmillan, 1969

36. Bacterial endocarditis, *Harrison's Principles of Internal
    Medicine*, Sixth edition, McGraw-Hill, 1970

37. Sexton et al, Surgery for left-sided native valve endocarditis, http://www.uptodate.com/contents/surgery-for-left-sided-native-valve-endocarditis

Just a Migraine:
38. Pineal Gland, https://en.wikipedia.org/wiki Pineal gland#Calcification

39. Pineal Gland, Harrison's Principles of Internal Medicine, Sixth edition, McGraw-Hill, 1970, http://www.shift.is/pineal-gland/

40. OPDIVO (nivolumab) for Metastatic Squamous Non-Small Cell Lung Cancer, http://www.cancertherapyadvisor.com/opdivo-nivolumab-for-metastatic-squamous- non-small-cell-lung-cancer/slideshow/2748/

Upset Stomach:
41. Tagamet, Wikipedia, http://www.wikipedia.org/

42. Do Germs Cause Cancer?, Forbes, http://www.forbes.com/global/1999/1115/0223102a.html

A Special Man:
43. Aloysius Alzheimer, http://en.wikipedia.org/wiki/Alois_Alzheimer
44. Alzheimer's Disease, http://en.wikipedia.org/wiki/Alzheimer's_disease

45. Alzheimer's Drugs, https://www.washingtonpost.com/national/health-science/

46. Alzheimer's Drugs - Fact and Fiction, http://www.alzcompend.info/?p=244

A Rocky Adventure:
47. Kidney stone, Wikipedia, https://en.wikipedia.org/wiki/Kidney_stone

48. Hospital medicine, Wikipedia, https://en.wikipedia.org/wiki/Hospital_medicine

A Bug Story:
49. Clapesattle, Helen, What Causes Cancer? *The Doctors Mayo*, Mayo Foundation, 1969, http://patient.info/health.com

50. Do germs cause cancer? - Forbes, http://www.forbes.com/global/1999/1115/0223102a.html

51. History of Vaccine Development,books.Google.com

52. Blaser, Martin, MD, *Missing Microbes*, Picador,2014

A Matter of Fat:
53. *Harrison's Principles of Internal Medicine*, Sixth edition, McGraw-Hill, 1970

54. William Enos, Jr., Korean Soldiers Study « Heart Attack Prevention, http://www.epi.umn.edu/cvdepi/study-synopsis/korean-soldiers-study/

55. Akira Endo (biochemist), Wikipedia, https://en.wikipedia.org/wiki/

56. Hughes, Sue, ENHANCE Negative, Medscape, January 14, 2008, http://www.medscape.com/viewarticle/568763

57. Briffa, John, M.D., Do statins save lives in essentially healthy people? (No), June 30, 2010, http://www.drbriffa.com/2010/06/30/do-statins-save-lives-in-essentially-healthy- people-no/

A Colossal Lie:
58. Archie Cochrane and his vision for evidence-based medicine, http:www.ncbi.nlm.nih.gov/pmc/articles/PMC2746659/

59. Welch, Gilbert and Mogielnicki, Juliana, Presumed Benefit: lessons from the American experience with marrow transplantation for breast cancer, BMJ 2002;324:1088, http://www.ncbi.nlm.nih.gov/pmc/articles/PMC1123033/

60. False Hope: Bone Marrow Transplantation for Breast Cancer, N Engl J Med 2007; 357:1059-1060

61. Breast Cancer Researcher Admits Falsifying Data, New York Times, February 5, 2000

62. Bezwoda 1985 Breast Cancer Transplant Study Fraudulent | Cancer Network http://www.cancernetwork.com/articles/bezwoda-1985-breast-cancer-transplant-study-fraudulent

An Aging World:
63. Nutrition and the Decline in Mortality since 1700: Some Preliminary Findings, http://www.nber.org/chapters/c9687

64. Life Expectancy, Our World in Data, http://ourworldindata.org/data/population-growth-vital-statistics/life-expectancy/

65. The First Measured Century: Timeline: Data - Mortality, http://www.pbs.org/fmc/timeline/dmortality.htm

66. Medicare (United States), https://en.wikipedia.org/wiki, Medicare_(United_States)

67. U.S. health plans have history of cost overruns, The Washington Times, November 18, 2009, www.washingtontimes.com/news/2009/nov/18

68. Total Medicaid Spending 2014, The Henry J. Kaiser Family Foundation, http://kff.org/medicaid/state-indicator/total-medicaid-spending/

69. Medicare Spending 2015, The Henry J. Kaiser Family Foundation, http://kff.org/medicare/fact-sheet/medicare-spending-and-financing-fact-sheet/

70. U.S. Healthcare Expenditure 1965-2015 graph, nihms 139759f1

71. Deaths in the United States, 2010,
http://www.cdc.gov/nchs/data/databriefs/db99.htm

White as Snow:
72. Red Cell Aplasia in Children, Archives of Disease in Children, 1979, 54, 263-267

73. Transient Erythroblastopenia of Childhood (TEC) | Pediatrics Clerkship | The University of Chicago,
https://pedclerk.bsd.uchicago.edu/page/transient-erythroblastopenia-childhood-tec

Peanut and Potato:
74. Idiopathic Intracranial Hypertension: Practice Essentials, Background, Pathophysiology,
http://emedicine.medscape.com/article/1214410-overview

Final Thoughts:
75. Bubbles, Babies and Biology: The Story of Surfactant,
http://www.fasebj.org/content/18/13/1624e.full

76. Editor In Chief Of World's Best Known Medical Journal: Half ...,May 16, 2015, www.collective-evolution.com/.../editor-in-chief-of-worlds-best-known-Peer review: a flawed process at the heart of science and journals, R. Smith, 2006, www.ncbi.nlm.nih.gov/.

77. US death rates 1700-2010,
https://books.google.com

The Deacon's Masterpiece:
78. Oliver Wendell Holmes,Sr., The Deacon's Masterpiece,
http://www.eldritchpress.org/owh/shay.html

79. Lienhard, John H., No. 1013: Oliver Wendell Holmes,
http://www.uh.edu/engines/epi1013.htm

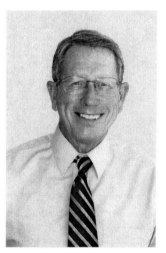

Doctor Ashcraft is a retired rural family physician and educator.
He and his wife Kay live in Billings, Montana.
They spend their time with their growing family, traveling,
volunteering, and pursuing hobbies.
They have three grown children and seven grandchildren.

CPSIA information can be obtained
at www.ICGtesting.com
Printed in the USA
FSOW01n2123010716
22303FS